MW00353789

Audiology in the USA

Audiology in the USA

James Jerger

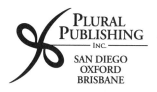

PLURAL
PUBLISHING
INC.

SAN DIEGO
OXFORD
BRISBANE

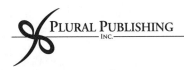

PLURAL PUBLISHING
INC.

5521 Ruffin Road
San Diego, CA 92123

e-mail: info@pluralpublishing.com
Web site: http://www.pluralpublishing.com

49 Bath Street
Abingdon, Oxfordshire OX14 1EA
United Kingdom

Copyright © by Plural Publishing, Inc. 2009

Typeset in 10½/13 Palatino by Flanagan's Publishing Services, Inc.
Printed in the United States of America by Bang Printing

All rights, including that of translation, reserved. No part of this publication may be reproduced, stored in a retrieval system, or transmitted in any form or by any means, electronic, mechanical, recording, or otherwise, including photocopying, recording, taping, Web distribution, or information storage and retrieval systems without the prior written consent of the publisher.

For permission to use material from this text, contact us by
Telephone: (866) 758-7251
Fax: (888) 758-7255
e-mail: permissions@pluralpublishing.com

Every attempt has been made to contact the copyright holders for material originally printed in another source. If any have been inadvertently overlooked, the publishers will gladly make the necessary arrangements at the first opportunity.

Library of Congress Cataloging-in-Publication Data:

Jerger, James.
  Audiology in the USA / James Jerger.
    p. ; cm.
  Includes bibliographical references and index.
  ISBN-13: 97-81-5975-6316-1 (alk. paper)
  ISBN-10: 1-5975-6316-1 (alk. paper)
 1. Audiology—United States—History. I. Title.
  [DNLM: 1. Audiology—history—United States WV 11 AA1 J55a 2008]
  RF291.J47 2008
  617.8—dc22

                                                    2008038403

CONTENTS

FOREWORD

Before you go any farther, read what Jim has written about me on page xiii in his Preface. There is an axiom in academia—"any book that cites my work in admiration is a fine publication worthy of worldwide distribution." So I must in all honesty ask that Jim Jerger's name be substituted for mine once again.

Why do I say "once again"? In December of 2002, Jim Jerger kindly came to LSU to applaud my career at a retirement party. To paraphrase this witty clever man, whom I have always admired from the beginning of our association, he said something like:

It is a pleasure and an honor to speak in glowing terms about a man whose influence on our field has been immeasurable, whose leadership and originality have set the stage for the development of a strong and powerful profession . . .

And as he went on and on, I muttered in a barely audible fashion "Jim that sounds much more like you than me." At the end of his encomium, he smiled and said " . . . But enough about me, we are here to celebrate Chuck's retirement."

No one laughed louder or longer than I did. It is to Jim we owe the popular acceptance of much of our modern audiologic practice differentiating cochlear from retrocochlear disease, starting with Békésy types, SISI, SPAR, tone decay, and so on and, of course, the ubiquitous test battery principle which now is the cornerstone of good audiology.

My honor, respect, and admiration for both Jim and Susan have only grown over the years. But it should come as no surprise that my view of our profession's history would have a slightly different twist based on discoveries made in intellectual streams quite different from those that formed the basis of audiology as Jim lived it. Other members of our profession were more strongly influenced by NIH and its training and research programs. Jim and Susan both played strong roles in promoting Audiology and its scientific validity in halls of NINDB and ultimately NIDCD. I daresay, without his support, some of my own grant applications would never have been approved.

Sadly, only a few of our audiologic colleagues have held NIH grants, but those who have, are leaders in our field and have published in the most prestigious journals in the world, including *Science* and *Nature*. Brenda Ryals of James Madison University, for example, published some of the germinal papers on hair cell regeneration and, working with Ed Rubel, helped discover that chicks regrow hair cells after noise trauma. That opened a remarkable chapter in auditory science, which uncovers new findings almost weekly.

Through my personal early postdoctoral training, underwritten by NIH, my notion of the first audiologists included C. C. Bunch. But I must add his anatomist-colleague-mentor Stacy Guild Ph.D. who learned about the WE 1-A from Bunch (or perhaps the other way around—history is unclear) and then rolled the first Western Electric audiometer around the wards of the Johns Hopkins, doing bedside audiograms on dying patients. He then collected their temporal bones and showed that high-frequency hearing loss (measured albeit tenuously to 16,384 Hz with Bakelite headphones!) was associated with loss of hair cells and nerve fibers at the basal turn of the cochlea. That publication dovetailed with von Békésy's first publication on traveling wave theory, meshed with Wever and Bray's findings on cochlear electrical events, and spawned immediate attempts to record human action potentials and cochlear microphonics instead of audiograms. The search for the objective audiogram had already begun before there were even norms or very many official practitioners. Their attempts to record these events from human ears unfortunately were technically premature, despite von Békésy's and Lempert's best efforts. Merle Lawrence, and later Joe Hawkins, were among the leaders who ushered in a new era of correlating electrically extracted audition with physiology and anatomy. This was the slightly different stream into which I fell as part of my early NIH-supported postdoctoral training. Without NIH support, I feel our field would have taken a somewhat less scientific turn.

It was one of my responsibilities as a postdoctoral fellow at the Johns Hopkins to test terminal patients bedside, get permission to harvest their temporal bones, and get the bones and fix them for subsequent study. It was there I first realized that what Jim and his colleagues already knew, that the pure tone audiogram did not always mesh with what textbooks taught about the underlying cochlear anatomy and physiology. My audiologic brain was expanding and people like Wever, Lawrence, Schuknecht, Lempert, and Guild, not to mention Ira Hirsh (none of whom would ever qualify for ASHA certification—sigh) were really teaching us important things about our patients from an entirely nonclinical perspective.

And Jim is, of course, also responsible in part for that expansion because he introduced me to, and captivated me with, the writings of Edward de Bono. (*The Five Day Course in Thinking* and *Serious Creativity* are two of my personal favorites.) Let me explain. de Bono taught us ways of thinking to address both the "quite impossible" and the "incredibly mundane" as worthy of some attention. So, in much of my teaching of medical students, neuroscientists, audiologists, and colleagues I ask the rhetorical question "Why Is the Sky Dark at Night?" The common and expected answer is: "Because the sun's on the other side of the earth." Well, that explains why the *earth* is dark at night, but why don't we see the light of the sun bypassing the earth on its way out to space? Is the earth casting a huge shadow that blocks out everything but somehow manages to skip the moon, the stars, and any planes or satellites passing by way up in the sky? Obviously not. The (partially) correct answer is that the sky is brilliantly lit with *infrared* light visible to cats, rats, mice, and so on but not to humans. The sun's light is moving away from us at the speed of light and undergoes a Doppler shift, which causes it to appear as infrared instead of visible spectrum light.

Why is this an important thinking exercise? We don't mull over this dark sky paradox because we have a logical answer that satisfies us, even though it is wrong. Once we make up an answer that satisfies us, we stop looking. The nature of the human brain is that we make up stories to fit the facts that we observe (cf. Gazzaniga and the *Ethical Brain*), which in turn dampens our curiosity.

For example, why do we have a middle ear muscle reflex and what does it have to do with the audiogram? We were taught (or taught each other) that it is a protective mechanism for "loud noises" and we elicit it with a loud sound to the ear. But virtually all mammals and many other species have such a reflex. Why would Nature (my apologies to the Intelligent Design folks) anticipate the industrial revolution and introduce a protective device that attenuates *low* frequencies by virtue of its increase in stiffness of the ossicular chain. In humans the middle ear muscle reflex is invoked 50 msec *in anticipation of* the onset of the voice, and in part as a protective device for the almost 115 dB SPL *low* frequencies generated in the vocal tract. In many mammals (bats, for example), it is a tool to modulate echo returns and keep them from impinging on pinging sounds emitted from the vocal tract.

I include this homily in honor of Jim and his contribution to our profession. He makes us think, and come up with new answers. What's more, his own relentless attempts to separate cochlear from retrocochlear disorders has an orderly interlaced lattice-like structure, which allows its ultimate reconfiguration once new facts are discovered.

Let me clarify. Because of the history of our profession and its reliance on the pure tone audiogram as a gold standard, we now have one of our most critical problems facing us. "If your only tool is a hammer, the whole world looks like a nail." Our primary tool was the pure tone audiogram and we thought that, once we obtained it, "our job was done." As Jim quite rightly notes in the text, some of our otolaryngology colleagues would like to relegate us to that role, or automate us out of our work. We must revise much of our thinking about the audiogram and learn instead to interpret it through modern concepts of physiology which we didn't have even 15 years ago.

To amplify, most of the work published in our journals views the ABR and middle ear muscle reflexes through the prism of the "getting the audiogram" or diagnosing a tumor, rather than the underlying physiology. In the late 1960s and early 1970s, Henry Spoendlin showed that it was the *inner hair cell* that mediated virtually all the auditory

nerve activity in mammals. So the audiogram, the middle ear muscle reflexes, the ABR, and all of our understanding of speech perception and the articulation index reviewed in this book that were championed by Harvey Fletcher et al. now have to be re-examined from the point of view of the integrity of the inner hair cell, its dynamic range of only 65 dB, and the synchrony of the nerve fibers which it subtends. People with nearly normal audiograms can in fact have no ABRs because they lack synchrony, and, similarly, people with very poor audiograms can have *normal emissions* because their inner hair cells and/or nerve fibers are not functioning well. These observations demand that we put the quest for the "objective audiogram" and "objective hearing measurement" in a different light.

David Kemp's discovery of otoacoustic emissions allows us to study the outer hair cell almost in isolation. We recognize the outer hair cell has a wide dynamic range cochlear amplifier and, therefore, in the presence of normal emissions, an additional hearing aid is certainly not physiologically called for in the selected frequency ranges. Thus, we as audiologists are the only profession that can noninvasively dissect the cochlea into inner and outer hair cell function in living humans, and manage them from a physiologic perspective rather than exclusively from their audiograms. Unfortunately, the two-stage test of emissions first, followed by ABR second, described here by Jim as a major achievement in our profession has to be re-examined in the light of recent findings. It should be ABR first, and emissions second, because almost 40% of NICU babies will have normal emissions and absent or abnormal EcochGs or ABRs. They will escape proper diagnosis and management (Rea & Gibson) if emissions are done first.

Outer hair cells can be tested with otoacoustic emissions and cochlear microphonics.

Inner hair cell integrity can be inferred from five test results: A synchronous N1 in the EcochG, a similarly synchronous Wave I in the ABR, recordable Summating potentials, brief cochlear microphonics (again because they come from *any* hair cell) and robust middle ear muscle reflexes at or less than 95 dB HL *regardless* of the audiogram. An absent reflex in the presence of normal emissions, or an absent ABR in the presence of normal emissions are cardinal signs of auditory neuropathy/dys-synchrony, a set of conditions that apply in at least 15% of our hearing-impaired children and many of our adults who are inexplicably poor hearing aid users or who have "dead zones" (Brian C. J. Moore).

With this armamentarium, why do we still fit hearing aids based on the audiogram without testing the underlying physiology? Because we think we know why the sky is dark at night and don't think beyond the pure tone audiogram the way Jim has always exhorted us to do. This is the core of a new way to look at audiology. It complements and plays a reprise to all of our audiologic forebearers, and ties together many loose ends which, at the time of original report, had only limited physiologic explanations.

By applying the Jerger and Hayes cross-check principle, we can study each new patient physiologically with tympanometry, reflexes, and emissions. This trio predicts what the audiologic results *should* be but prevents us from viewing the audiogram as the gold standard of hearing. The same audiogram can lead to entirely different auditory perceptions when and if inner hair cells and/or nerve fibers are disabled. Therefore, "fixing or compensating for the audiogram," as suggested by many of our forebearers is appropriate only if the outer hair cells and, in part, the cochlear battery (endocochlear potential) are the culprits.

When inner hair cells and/or nerve fibers underlie the poor audiogram (and sometimes their accompanying audiograms can be nearly normal!), we have an entirely new way to classify their problems. What looks like auditory processing disorder (APD) may really be cases of auditory neuropathy/auditory dys-synchrony (AN/AD), with nearly normal audiograms, poor hearing in noise, and poor performance on the SCAN or any of the dichotic procedures commonly applied to make the APD diagnosis. It is here that assistive technologies, which essentially enhance the signal-to-noise ratio become our strongest weapons. Inner hair cell and nerve fiber losses, often revealed by extraordinarily poor hearing in noise scores, ultimately will yield to FM enhancement, assistive listening devices (ALDs), or cochlear implants, provided the impairment does not stem from thalamic, cerebellar, or cortical impairment. C.C. Bunch's patient, whom Jim thought might have Ménière's disease, could just as easily have had temperature-sensitive auditory neuropathy/dys-synchrony. But the advent of anything that enhances signal-to-noise ratio can just as easily be viewed in the context of ameliorating inner hair cell and nerve fiber loss.

So the six streams of audiology that Jim has so elegantly outlined in this book all will converge in the future on the underlying physiology and genetics of our patients.

Why genetics?

Within the next few years, chips will be available that can sample droplets of blood from our patients and tell us whether they are homozygous or heterozygous for many different genetic forms of deafness. (See http://webh01.ua.ac.be/hhh/ for almost daily updates on the status of genes and deafness.) Knowing the underlying genetic causes of various types of hearing loss will liberate us from categorizing hearing loss as simply "conductive or sensorineural." We will certainly be able to understand and better manage the underlying mechanisms of various hearing losses and both apply and develop new tools for assessment. The most important tools of the future will be both genetic and physiologic, especially if we can develop a noninvasive or nondestructive method for evaluating the endocochlear potential in humans. Knowing the status of the cochlear battery will open new vistas for both diagnosis and management.

So, in summary, my favorite audiologist of all time, the man in our field I hold in the greatest of respect, has brought us to a place where we can liberate ourselves from the search for the all elusive Holy Grail of the *audiogram*. We can now amend all of our practices with physiologic and mechanistic underpinnings to better treat our patients and work with our professional colleagues to better understand some of the mysteries we encounter.

We certainly cannot say that once we "get the pure tone audiogram," we now know all there is to know about Why the (audiologic) Sky Is Dark at Night, Jim Jerger has helped us reach a new place, a new promised land, where we have all the "hallmarks of a robust and growing profession with a remarkable history."

Charles Berlin, Ph.D.

Reference

Rea, P. A., & Gibson, W. P. (2003). Evidence for surviving inner hair cell function in congenitally cleat ears. *Laryngoscope, 113*(11), 2030–2034.

PREFACE

In this small volume, I have attempted to describe the major historical highlights of the profession of audiology in America over the past half century and to trace the divergent paths that specialization has followed as the profession matured. This was certainly a daunting task, but I have had the privilege of having been present at many of the landmark events marking the progress of the profession. And I have been able to draw on the recollections of many of my contemporaries over the years, especially my fellow student and steadfast friend, Earl Harford. As graduate students at Northwestern University in the early 1950s, we were fortunate to study under, and later work with, many of the people who shaped our profession in its infancy, Harold Westlake, Raymond Carhart, Helmer Myklebust, and John Gaeth.

Throughout the past half century, moreover, I have been privileged to interact with a number of outstanding otolaryngology colleagues; first George Shambaugh, John Ballenger, and Eugene Derlacki at Northwestern University, later Bobby Alford at Baylor College of Medicine, and more recently Gail Neely of Washington University in St. Louis and George Gates of the University of Washington. All have had a positive influence on my own work over the years.

I have been fortunate to know, over the past 50 years, most of the leading figures in audiology, but the one individual whom I hold in unique esteem is Charles Berlin, for many years leader of the Kresge Research Laboratory of the South at the Louisiana State University School of Medicine in New Orleans, and now carrying on his impressive research and inspired teaching at the University of South Florida. To my mind, no one better exemplifies the qualities of imagination, research rigor, and clinical investigation that have provided the foundation for, and the successful growth of, audiology throughout the second half of the 20th century.

I have benefited immeasurably from the many students I have mentored over the years; at Northwestern, Robert Harrison, John Peterson, and Laszlo Stein; at Baylor College of Medicine, John Allen, Denice Brown, Robert Fifer, James Hall III, Maureen Hannley, Deborah Hayes, Susan Jerger, Karen Johnson, Craig Jordan, William Keith, Henry Lew, Brad Stach, Lois Sutton, and Ann Thompson; at the University of Texas/Dallas, Rebecca Estes, Ralf Greenwald, Jeffrey Martin, Deborah Moncrieff, Gail Tillman, Ilse Wambacq, Tara Reed, Jyutika Mehta, and Gary Overson.

I am particularly indebted, in this work, to Cynthia Compton Conley, whose comprehensive knowledge and expertise in hearing assistance technology (HAT) has been of immeasurable assistance.

But the single individual most responsible for the completion of this work is my companion and helpmate for the past 45 years, my wife Susan Jerger, whose wise counsel and assistance have sustained me over this long audiologic journey.

Amassing all of the information in this book, especially details of the various military programs, the VA program, and the various professional organizations has required the active cooperation of many friends and colleagues. I am particularly indebted to John

Allen, James Battey, Lucille Beck, Jon Belgique, Moe Bergman, Charles Berlin, Cynthia Compton Conley, Kyle Dennis, John Ferraro, Vic Gladstone, Gretchen Haywood, Earl Harford, James Henry, Celia Hooper, Susan Jerger, Angela Loavenbruck, Craig Newman, Glen Rovig, Brad Stach, Brian Walden, Laura Ann Wilber, and Richard Wilson.

It should be noted that this book represents a substantial expansion of a book chapter, entitled "A Brief History of Audiology in the United States," originally prepared for a textbook, *Audiology: Science to Practice* edited by Steve Kramer. I am indebted to Steve, and to Plural Publishing, Inc., for permission to expand that chapter into this book. Additionally, the section on auditory processing disorder is an expansion of a chapter prepared for a book, *Current Controversies in Central Auditory Processing Disorder (CAPD)*, edited by Anthony Cacace and Dennis McFarland, and included with their permission.

Finally, in a single volume like this, it is not possible to include all of the important contributions that audiologists have made to their profession. There is just not enough space. Regretably, I have had to be selective. I sincerely hope that those individuals whose work has been omitted will understand the constraints and limitations imposed upon such an enterprise.

James Jerger, Ph.D.

This book is dedicated to the memory of Raymond Carhart, of Northwestern University; truly the father of audiology.

SECTION I

The Early Years

It is certainly the case that many 19th and early 20th century scientists and otolaryngologists, especially in Germany, laid the groundwork for the profession of audiology, as they developed procedures for the evaluation of hearing loss, based largely on the use of tuning forks. Prominent among these were Ernst Weber (1795–1878), famous for the Weber test for differentiating unilateral conductive from unilateral sensory neural loss, Heinrich Rinne (1819–1868) who developed the Rinne tuning fork test for differentiating conductive from sensory neural loss, and Marie Gellé (1834–1923) who devised a test for stapes fixation, anticipating tympanometry by several decades. Further elaboration of these important early contributions can be found in the monograph, *A History of Audiology* by Harald Feldmann, published in 1970 in the Beltone Translations series by the Beltone Institute for Hearing Research; but the history of modern audiology in the United States begins in 1922 with the design and fabrication of the first commercial audiometer, the Western Electric 1-A, by Harvey Fletcher and R. L. Wegel.

1

The Pioneers

Harvey Fletcher (Figure 1–1) was one of the true pioneers of research in speech communication. After teaching physics for five years at Brigham Young University in Provo, Utah, Fletcher moved to New York to carry out research in sound at the Western Electric Company. Here he participated in the development of the Western Electric hearing aid, the first to employ vacuum tubes; the initial model was delivered to none other than Thomas A. Edison. Harvey Fletcher's book *Speech and Hearing* for many years was the accepted standard guiding research in speech communication. As director of physical research at the Bell Telephone Laboratories in New Jersey, Fletcher set the stage for what later became the concept of the articulation index, and, more recently, the speech intelligibility index. He helped to found, and served as first president of, the Acoustical Society of America.

The Western Electric 1-A audiometer was quite large by today's standards and fairly expensive ($1500.00). As Figure 1–2 shows, it was hardly portable, but a later model, the WE 2-A, was smaller and lighter. It was sold mainly for use in otolaryngology practices. Within two years the Sonotone Jones-Knudson Model 1, became commercially available. Otolaryngologists were the primary users of audiometers in the 1920s and 1930s. Their enthusiasm was tempered, however, by the fact that there was no common standard for calibrating the devices. Each manufacturer relied on its own laboratory data, usually based on results from a few people available around the laboratory. Thus, the same patient might show somewhat different losses on two different audiometers. The problem was that no one was quite sure what were the SPL levels corresponding to average normal hearing in the population.

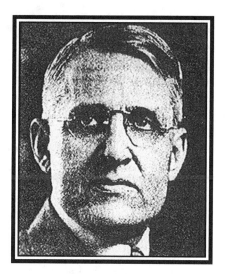

Figure 1–1. Harvey Fletcher.

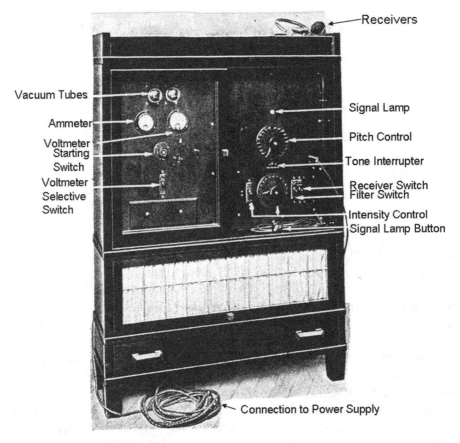

Figure 1–2. The Western Electric Model 1-A audiometer.

The Saga of Average Normal Hearing

In 1935 The United States Public Health Service (USPHS) undertook a fairly massive effort for the time, a survey of hearing sensitivity in the United States. Willis Beasley, a public health officer, was appointed to carry out the survey during the years 1935-1936; in subsequent years it became known as the "Beasley survey." Considering that no one had ever undertaken such a study before, the planning, execution, and reporting were remarkably sophisticated. The SPL levels obtained by the Beasley survey provided, for the first time, large-sample data defining average normal hearing over the frequency range from 128 Hz to 8192 Hz.

The first standard for the calibration of audiometers in the United States was published in 1951 by the American Standards Association, a voluntary group of consumers, manufacturers, engineers, and specialists. The sound pressure levels (SPL) values from the Beasley survey corresponding to average normal hearing at each test frequency (the zero HTL line on the audiogram) became, in 1951, the basis for the calibration of all audiometers in the United States. And, because no other country had undertaken a similar survey, the ASA-1951 standard (which came to be known as the "American standard") was adopted by many other countries as the basis for calibrating their audiometers. But in the early 1950s two other hearing surveys were carried out, one in the United Kingdom (UK), the other in Japan. The two surveys were in agreement: both found average normal hearing to be about 10 dB better than the American standard. In an effort to understand what might account for the approximately 10-dB discrepancy between the ASA-51 and the UK findings, the Research Center of the Subcommittee on Noise in Industry, in Los Angeles, authorized Aram Glorig to plan and execute another survey of average normal hearing in which the exact methods and procedures employed in the Beasley survey would be carefully repeated. Audiometers and audiometric booths were set up at the Wisconsin State Fair in 1954, and 3500 fairgoers were tested audiometrically. Results essentially replicated the Beasley findings. This prompted Glorig to go back to the Wisconsin State Fair, in 1955, and carry out another survey, but using what he termed "laboratory methodology," in which threshold was crossed at least three times in each direction. This time results were about 10 dB better, and in agreement with the UK/Japan results. Glorig concluded that the difference lay in the technique of threshold determination. Apparently, the difference between, on the one hand, the Beasley and 1954 Wisconsin State Fair results, and on the other hand the UK/Japan and the 1955 Wisconsin State Fair results, could best be attributed to better audiometric testing technique. It seemed that experience over the period from the 1930s to the 1950s, especially as a result of World War II military programs, had improved threshold seeking technique, resulting in more accurate threshold estimates.

After a good many international meetings, checks, and counterchecks on possible procedural and/or calibration microphone, earphone, and coupler differences, and many other possible reasons for the discrepancy, all finally agreed, in an international meeting at Rapallo, Italy, that the International Standards Organization (ISO) should issue, in 1964, a new standard that all could agree on. This became known as the ISO-64 standard. It was essentially based on the findings of the UK and Japan surveys. From that point on, audiometers worldwide could be calibrated to the same standard.

This change in the basis for calibrating the zero HTL line on the audiogram had a major impact on a number of agencies in this country, particularly the military and the Veterans Administration. Because compensation for service-induced hearing loss was based on audiometric hearing threshold levels, a change of the zero loss level of 10 dB, had the potential to increase compensation benefits nationwide to a financially alarming degree. There was a long transition period during which reporting degree of hearing loss in the United States required that the calibration standard of the particular audiometer used for the measurement (ASA-51 or ISO-64) be reported as well. Eventually, however, all of these problems were resolved. Later, in 1969, the ASA (newly renamed the American National Standards Institute [ANSI]), made some minor adjustment to the ISO-64 standard, resulting in the ANSI-69 standard, and still later the ANSI-96 standard, which is now the basis for the calibration of audiometers in the United States. Although other details of these standards have changed slightly over the years, the ISO-64 SPL levels have remained virtually unchanged.

The Audiogram Recording Form

The year 1922 also saw the design of what we now know as the pure-tone audiogram recording form. It was conceived jointly by

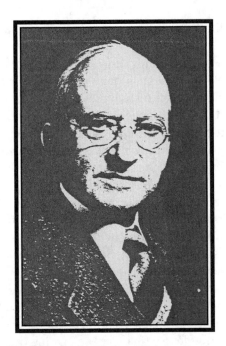

Figure 1–3. Edmund Prince Fowler.

The First Audiologist

The first genuine audiologist in the United States was undoubtedly Cordia C. Bunch. As a graduate student at the University of Iowa, late in the World War I, Bunch came under the influence of Carl Seashore, a psychologist who was studying the measurement of musical aptitude, and Lee Wallace Dean, an otolaryngologist. Together they convinced Bunch to undertake a five-year project on the practical application of methods for testing hearing. Because audiometers were not yet available commercially, Bunch developed his own instrument, called the "pitch range audiometer." It covered the frequency range from 30 to 10,000 Hz and intensities capable of reaching threshold in one direction and pain in the other. With this audiometer, Bunch plotted what he called the "hearing fields" of Dean's patients, from thresholds of hearing to thresholds of discomfort.

scientists Fletcher and Wegel and by an otolaryngologist, Edmund Prince Fowler (Figure 1–3) of Columbia University, the latter one of the great pioneers of otologic medicine. Unfortunately, they made two decisions that have continued to haunt us for the past 50 years. First, they proposed that "hearing loss" at each test frequency be expressed relative to "average normal hearing," a sound pressure level (SPL) that varies with frequency. Second, they thought that degree of loss ought to be plotted downward on the graph. All of this probably seemed like a good idea at the time, but it has caused unremitting problems in relating the audiogram to the performance of amplification devices, where performance at each frequency is expressed relative to a common SPL reference and is plotted upward on the graph in conformity with standard scientific practice. But at this point the practice is so ingrained that all efforts to bring reason to the situation have failed utterly.

After obtaining his Ph.D. degree, Bunch stayed on briefly at Iowa, then moved for a short time to Johns Hopkins University, as Associate in Research Otology. In the meantime, L. W. Dean had moved from the University of Iowa to Washington University in St. Louis and invited Bunch to rejoin him there. Bunch accepted and was appointed Professor of Applied Physics of Otology at the Washington University School of Medicine. For the next two decades Bunch gathered a massive number of air-conduction audiograms on Dean's patients, analyzed them, and wrote up his findings. Over the years from 1919 to 1943, Bunch published papers covering an astonishing range of topics. He wrote on the use of the audiometer, the importance of measuring sensitivity in the range of frequencies above the conventional audiometric range, the effect of age on audiometric thresholds, occupational and traumatic deafness, traumatic loss from firecracker explosion, progression of loss in otosclerosis, deafness in aviators, conservation of hearing in industry, hearing aids, race and sex variations in hearing thresholds, otitis media, effect of removal of one entire cerebral hemisphere, calculating percentage of loss for medicolegal purposes, and the effect of absence of the organ of Corti on the audiogram.

Bunch carried out the first systematic studies of the relation between types of hearing loss and audiometric patterns. These pioneering efforts were published in 1943 in a slender volume entitled *Clinical Audiometry*, which is now a classic in the field. The title page is shown in Figure 1–4. One case study from the book illustrates how his insights

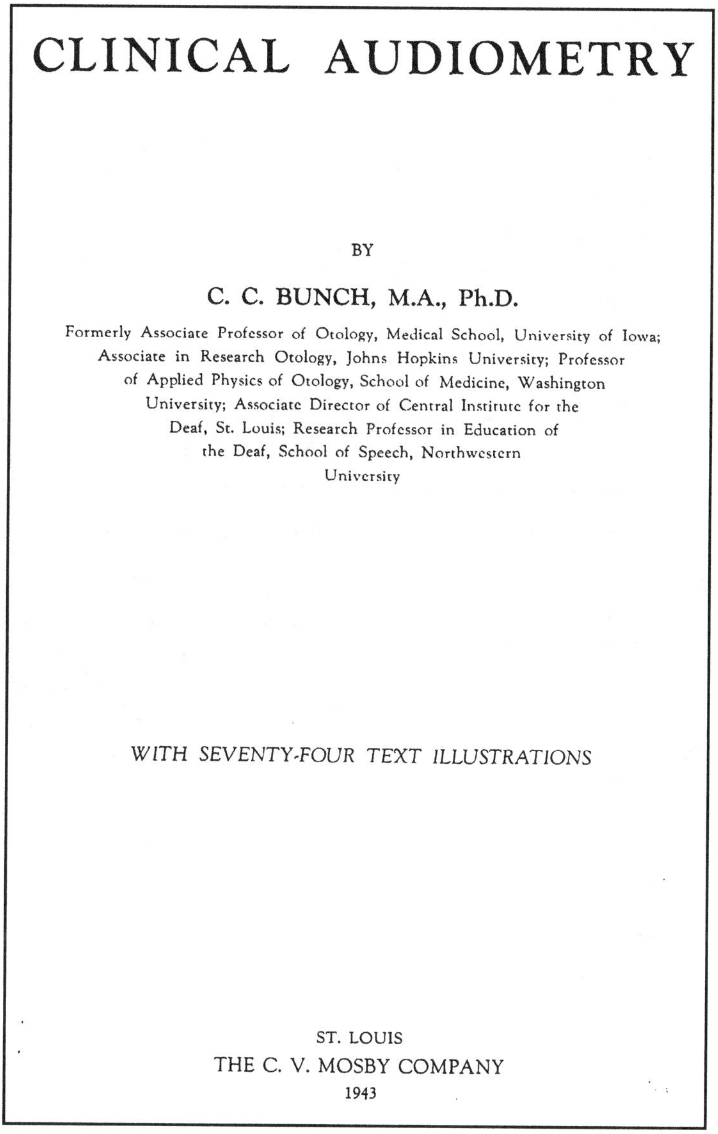

CLINICAL AUDIOMETRY

BY

C. C. BUNCH, M.A., Ph.D.

Formerly Associate Professor of Otology, Medical School, University of Iowa; Associate in Research Otology, Johns Hopkins University; Professor of Applied Physics of Otology, School of Medicine, Washington University; Associate Director of Central Institute for the Deaf, St. Louis; Research Professor in Education of the Deaf, School of Speech, Northwestern University

WITH SEVENTY-FOUR TEXT ILLUSTRATIONS

ST. LOUIS
THE C. V. MOSBY COMPANY
1943

Figure 1–4. The title page of C. C. Bunch's classic volume, *Clinical Audiometry*, published by C. V. Mosby in 1943.

foreshadowed ideas that did not come to fruition until many years later. In the book he presents the audiogram of a 42-year-old man with what may very well have been Ménière's disease (Figure 1–5).

Bunch noted that the audiogram may not always help in the selection of a hearing aid and, indeed, may even lead to the wrong recommendation. In this case, he advised an aid with uniform frequency response, but subsequent evaluation showed that the patient understood very little in spite of the amplification afforded by the aid. Then he tried a Y-cord arrangement to both ears, but the patient could still understand very little. At this point, he began to suspect that something was out of order. He returned to the audiometer, presented tones at suprathreshold levels, and simply asked the patient to make pitch comparisons of the tones. Using this procedure he discovered that tones at 128, 256, and 512 Hz all were heard at the appropriate pitch and in the proper order, but that tones at frequencies of 1024, 1448, 2048, and 2896 Hz "all sounded alike and lacked tonal quality." Bunch speculated that the hearing aid was useful only in the low frequency range below 512 Hz, but of little value in the frequency region important for understanding speech. Bunch then made the prescient observation that, if it had been possible to administer simple speech audiometric testing, then the discrepancy between the audiogram and the patient's actual ability to understand speech could have been detected and the patient would not have had to go to the expense of purchasing a hearing aid that was not very helpful.

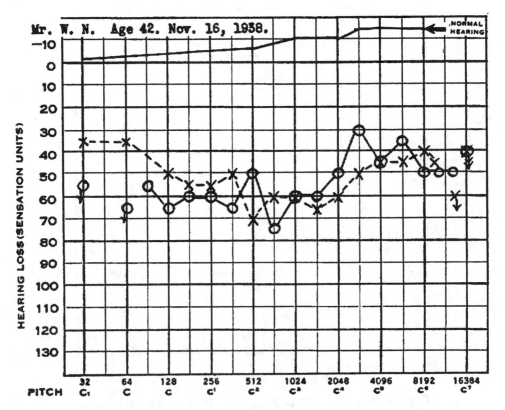

Figure 1–5. Audiogram of a Bunch patient who fared poorly with hearing aids.

Here, we can almost see the thinking of the consummate clinician/investigator at work. With only the pure-tone, air-conduction audiometer as test equipment, he senses a puzzling disagreement between his test results and the patient's ability to function with amplification. Determined to explore the matter, he does rudimentary pitch comparisons and discovers that all tones above 512 Hz have lost tonal pitch quality. He speculates that this may be the result of a unique aural pathology of which he is apparently unaware. He speculates that standardized speech audiometric tests, which, of course, were not available in 1938, would have been helpful in identifying the problem and thereby avoiding an inappropriate hearing aid fitting.

Bunch was probably the first to suggest that, in seeking threshold, the tonal stimulus should be keyed on and off rather than left on continuously, the first to suggest that testing should begin at 1000 Hz, and the first to suggest that total unilateral malingering would be revealed by the absence of an appropriate "shadow curve" on the presumably deaf ear.

After Dean's retirement, Bunch briefly became Associate Director of the Central Institute for the Deaf in St. Louis. In 1941 he accepted an offer from the School of Speech at Northwestern University to come to Evanston as Research Professor in Education of the Deaf, and to teach courses in hearing testing and hearing disorders. There he met and did a bit of mentoring of a young faculty member in speech science, Raymond Carhart. In June of 1942 Bunch unexpectedly died at the age of 57. In order to proceed with the course, the NU administration tapped Carhart to teach Bunch's courses. And the rest, as they say, is history. Carhart told me, years later, that no single person had had more influence on his career than C. C. Bunch.

2

Origins of the Words "Audiology" and "Audiologist"

The late Kenneth Berger, of Kent State University, dug deeply into the origin of the word "audiology." His 1976 report details the several claims and counterclaims surrounding the first use of the word. He reports that the earliest claim was made by a New York City dentist, Dr. Mayer B. A. Schier. According to Berger, Scheir claimed that he coined the words "audiology" and "auditology" in 1935, but the claim did not appear in print until 1950. Another claim, according to Berger, arose from an organization called the "Auricular Foundation Institute of Audiology." Two individuals, William B. Hargrave and M. E. Trainor asserted, in 1953, that their organization had developed, as early as 1939, the first course in "Audiological Problems in Education," which was offered at Claremont College in California. Hargrave claimed that the word "audiology" was used in that course as early as 1942. In that same year, according to Hargrave, an organization called the California Audiological Society attracted students from many of California's colleges and universities. Berger notes, however, that he was unable to find documentary evidence of any of this before 1948.

Berger's research unearthed yet another interesting claim. In 1939 Stanley Nowak and J. Fran Stengel formed the Telephonics Company which made the Telephonics 38

and 39 earphones for use in communication devices by the United States Navy. The Telephonics TDH-39 earphone became, for many years thereafter, the earphone of choice for audiometers and for psychoacoustic research. Telephonics employee Sterling J. Sears, an engineer, developed a hearing aid to be marketed by a related firm, called Telephonics Laboratories of America. To assist in the marketing of this aid, Stanley Nowak prepared a training manual for distributors entitled "Telephonics Primer and Fitting Manual." In this manual, Nowak is said to have introduced, in 1939, the term "Telephonics Audiologist"; the term was used in hearing aid marketing as early as 1940 by Andy Harvey who became a distributor of Maico hearing aids. Shortly thereafter, however, Harvey was discouraged from using the term "audiologist" by Leland Watson, president of Maico, who felt that the term should not be used by hearing aid dealers.

It is not known whether any of this early use of the terms "audiology" and "audiologist" in the hearing aid industry were known by individuals in otolaryngology or in the academic areas associated with aural rehabilitation, but three individuals in those areas, Norton Canfield, an otolaryngologist at Yale University, Hallowell Davis, an auditory scientist at Central Institute for the

Deaf, and Raymond Carhart, a professor at Northwestern University, claimed to have originated the term independently. It is not certain which of these three individuals was the person actually responsible for first suggesting the term. At one time or another, each claimed to have been the progenitor. At the Second International Conference in Audiology, held in London in 1950, Canfield gave a speech in which he claimed to have been the first to use the word "audiology" in 1945 at the dedication of a plaque honoring Walter Hughson at the Deshon General Hospital in Butler, Pennsylvania. Neither Davis nor Carhart laid claim to an earlier date.

Berger reports that the first use of the words "audiology" or "audiologist" in printed form that he was able to locate appeared in the *Journal of Speech Disorders* in 1946 in the form of a brief announcement that the "Speech Clinic at the U.S. Naval Hospital, Philadelphia, is the permanent Naval center for rehabilitation and for research in speech and Audiology." Also in 1946 the *Volta Review* reported that "Northwestern University, at Evanston, in its School of Speech offers a wide variety of courses in audiology leading to the degree of Bachelor of Science, Doctor of Philosophy and Doctor of Education."

In 1946 the Committee on the Conservation of Hearing of the American Academy of Ophthalmology and Otolaryngology (AAOO) recommended that training programs for audiologists be established in various universities and that the word "audiology" be recognized by the Academy. They suggested, further, that the Academy set up a bureau to "certificate and regulate" audiologists. This remains, up to the present, a contentious issue between audiologists and otolaryngologists (see Chapter 11, the Medical Connection).

The council of the American Speech Correction Association met late in 1947 and voted to include reference to hearing in the name of the association and in its journal but avoided the term "Audiology." Shortly thereafter the name was changed to the American Speech and Hearing Association (ASHA); its learned journal was changed from the *Journal of Speech Disorders* to the *Journal of Speech and Hearing Disorders*. In 1960 the ASHA created a new publication, the *Journal of Speech and Hearing Research*, which is still published under the title of *Journal of Speech, Language and Hearing Research*. Beginning in the early 1950s, ASHA broadened its certification program for speech pathologists to include separate certification requirements for audiologists.

By 1951 the term "audiology" was in such common usage that the highly respected and influential *Consumer Reports* carried an article on hearing and hearing aids in which it recommended that individuals seek the services of an audiology clinic. In that same year, 1951, in an article by George Shambaugh and Raymond Carhart, in the *Archives of Otolaryngology*, a brief historical note declared that the word audiology was coined in 1945 by Canfield, and independently by Carhart at the same time. But there is no documentation of either claim.

Hallowell Davis was perhaps the first to commit to print a formal definition of the term "audiology." In 1947 he defined audiology as "a general field of knowledge and of social endeavor centering around hearing," and suggested that the word "audiology" might be a useful name for the field even though linguists might not approve of adding a Greek suffix to a Latin root.

In 1949 Norton Canfield, published a short monograph entitled *Audiology: the Science of Hearing: A Developing Professional Specialty*. His definition of audiology was somewhat more inclusive, embracing not only the medical aspects of ear disease but the propagation and transmission of sound to the ear, all of the processes involved in its perception within the auditory system, the psychological processes invoked in the central interpretation of the sound, and the ultimate reaction of the listener.

In the same book Canfield, outlined the makeup of the audiology center of the future. His concept, illustrated in Figure 2–1, included almost every medical specialty except gynecology. A somewhat less ambitious version of this comprehensive concept was actually attempted in a small number of locales, including the Bill Wilkerson Center in Nashville and the Callier Center in Dallas. None have been able to maintain the full scope of Canfield's original vision, but the Wilkerson Center, under the initial leadership of Freeman McConnell and its subsequent development by Fred Bess (Figure 2–2), and the Callier Center, under the early leadership of Aram Glorig and more recent leadership of Ross Roeser (Figure 2–3), have become centers that meet the spirit, if not the letter, of Canfield's vision.

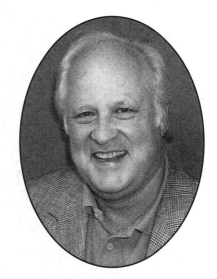

Figure 2–2. Fred Bess.

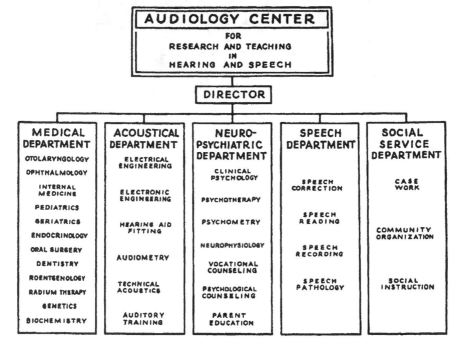

Figure 2–1. Canfield's concept of the makeup of an ideal Audiology Center.

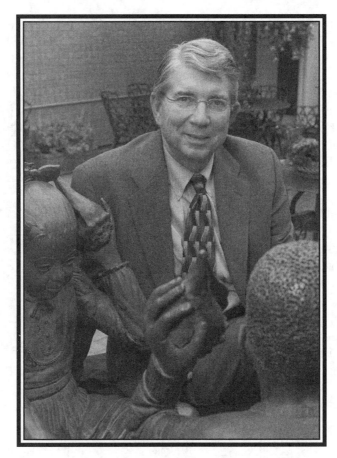

Figure 2–3. Ross Roeser.

3

The Military Programs During and After World War II

The profession owes a good deal to the military aural rehabilitation programs instituted by the United States Army and the Navy during the last two years of World War II. Although the army had established a hearing rehabilitation program at the Army General Hospital in Cape May, New Jersey, during World War I, services in that pre-amplification era were necessarily limited to lip reading training; the program serviced only 108 soldiers. But, by World War II, the wearable hearing aid was a reality, so that a broader range of services could be offered. In 1943 the U.S. Army set up three aural rehabilitation programs; one at the Borden General Hospital in Chickasha, Oklahoma, a second at the Hoff General Hospital in Santa Barbara, California, and a third at the Walter Reed General Hospital in Washington, DC. The Walter Reed program was shortly moved, however, to the Deshon General Hospital in Butler Pennsylvania. Early in 1944, the U.S. Navy organized its own aural rehabilitation center at the U.S. Naval hospital in Philadelphia. Two members of the staff at Hoff General Hospital, Second Lieutenants. Moe Bergman and Ira Hirsh, went on to distinguished careers in the field, Bergman at Hunter College of the City University of New York (CUNY) and later Tel Aviv University,

and Hirsh at Central Institute for the Deaf. Three staff members at the Borden General Hospital, Grant Fairbanks, Louis DiCarlo, and John Duffy, moved on after the war, to develop teaching and research programs at the University of Illinois, Syracuse University, and Brooklyn College, respectively. The Navy program at Philadelphia gave us three early leaders of the profession, William Hardy, Miriam Pauls, and Harriet Haskins, all of whom went on to make significant contributions at the Johns Hopkins University, especially in the evaluation of children.

But it was the acoustics unit at the Deshon Hospital that was to play perhaps the most influential role in the development of audiology as we know it today. Raymond Carhart (Figure 3–1) was assigned to head the acoustics unit at Deshon General hospital in Butler, Pennsylvania, first in a civil service position, later at the military rank of Captain. Although Carhart initiated an ambitious auditory training program, his principal rehabilitative weapon was the hearing aid, then a fairly bulky device about the size of a package of cigarettes, which was worn in the pocket or in a holder suspended around the neck. It was connected by a thin wire to a transducer mounted in a fully occluding earmold. Carhart's task was to devise a set

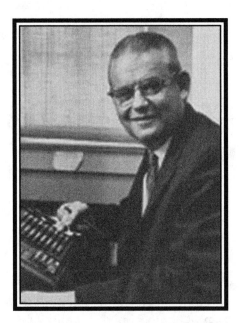

Figure 3–1. Raymond Carhart.

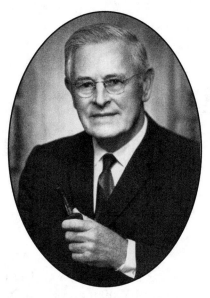

Figure 3–2. Hallowell Davis. (Courtesy of CID-Central Institute for the Deaf, St. Louis, MO.)

of procedures upon which to base a rational decision about which of several possible hearing aids should be dispensed to the serviceman. To accomplish this, Carhart virtually invented, from scratch, what we now know as speech audiometry. He adapted the earlier work at the Harvard Psychoacoustic Laboratory on spondee and phonemically balanced (PB) word lists into the concepts of the speech reception threshold (SRT), and the maximum PB score (PBmax). Two members of Carhart's staff at Deshon, Sgt. Fran Sonday and Pfc. Leo Doerfler, were destined for future fame in the profession, Sonday at the Indiana University Medical Center and Doerfler at the University of Pittsburgh.

During World War II, Hallowell Davis (Figure 3–2), then at Harvard University, conducted ground-breaking research on the effects of high noise levels on the auditory system. He was also instrumental in the preparation of the now famous "Harvard Report" in which a master hearing aid was used to study the extent to which matching the frequency response of the aid to a patient's audiometric contour was efficacious. Immediately after the war, Davis moved from Harvard to the Central Institute for the Deaf (CID) in St. Louis and collaborated with CID Director Richard Silverman on the book, *Hearing and Deafness: A Guide for Laymen*, which brought together much of what had been learned at the Aural Rehabilitation Centers during the war.

Shortly after the war's end, in September of 1946, the three Army Aural Rehabilitation units were closed. Hearing rehabilitation continued in a single center, the Army Audiology and Speech Center (AASC), located at the Forest Glen campus of the Walter Reed Army Medical Center in Washington, DC. Here it was to remain for 32 years until it was moved to Walter Reed's main campus in 1978. Over the period from 1971 to 2007, the audiologic research program at Walter Reed was ably directed by Brian Walden (Figure

3–3), assisted over the years by Robert Prosek, Allen Montgomery, Dan Schwartz, Sue Erdman, David Hawkins, David Fabry, Marjorie Leek, Ken Grant, Van Summers, Mary Cord, Therese Walden, and many temporary appointees. Under Walden's tutelage, the AASC research program made an impressive list of research contributions both to our basic understanding of hearing processes and to the efficacy of a number of intervention strategies.

The Army audiology program was also instrumental in training officers who went on to distinguished audiologic careers in civilian life. Chief among these were Don Worthington, Jerry Northern, Roy Sedge, Rodney Atack, Richard Danielson, David Chandler, Donald Bender, Ernest Hepler, Richard Dennis, Harvey Abrams, and Gus Mueller.

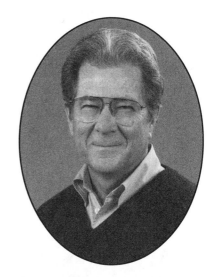

Figure 3–3. Brian Walden. (Courtesy of Sean M. Brennan.)

4

The VA Program

The profession of audiology owes a great debt to the program in audiology and speech pathology initiated by the Veterans Administration (VA), now the Department of Veterans Affairs. The VA programs have contributed to the training of future leaders of the profession, to leadership in developing models for the dispensing of amplification devices, and to the provision of excellent clinical services, and are moving to the forefront of audiologic research.

At the end of World War II, the army and navy continued scaled down versions of the wartime effort in seeing to the aural rehabilitation needs of their own personnel, but it became clear that caring for the vast majority of returning servicemen and servicewomen with hearing disorders would fall on the shoulders of the Veterans Administration. To plan for this daunting task, the VA's chief medical director appointed Norton Canfield, as a consultant. His task was to establish services for veterans that would continue the pattern set by the wartime military programs. Canfield set up what became known as the audiology and speech correction services under VA's Medical Rehabilitation Service. In 1946 Edward Truex, an otolaryngologist who had served as medical director at the Deshon Hospital, where Raymond Carhart had headed the acoustics department, was appointed as the first head of the

VA program. He was succeeded by Aram Glorig, another otolaryngologist, who went on to design, build, and initially direct the Callier Center for Communication Sciences and Disorders in Dallas, Texas. Merle Ansberry followed Glorig in the VA director's post until 1954, when he made an enviable move to head the program at the University of Hawaii in Honolulu. Ansberry was succeeded by Kenneth O. Johnson, former head of the VA service in San Francisco. Johnson convinced the Veterans Administration that functional hearing loss (pseudohypoacusis) was a serious problem and instituted a comprehensive testing program, which set the standard for functional evaluation for many years to come. Johnson also set into motion a 10-year review of all of the VA's compensation cases, resulting in substantial savings to the VA in compensation costs. Kenneth Johnson left the VA in 1956 to become executive secretary of ASHA, serving that organization ably until his retirement in 1980. From 1956 to 1980 the VA program was headed by Bernard Anderman, who had previously headed the New York VA service. Anderman was succeeded by Henry Spuehler, and Alan Boysen. The program is currently directed by Lucille Beck (Figure 4–1).

The first VA Audiology Clinic was established at the New York Regional Office in 1946. An exhaustive description of its

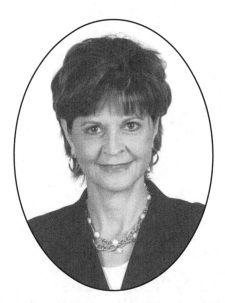

Figure 4–1. Lucille Beck. (Courtesy of Washington, DC Veterans Affairs Medical Center.)

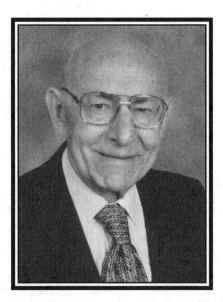

Figure 4–2. Moe Bergman. (Courtesy of Farag Peri.)

physical features and the services offered can be found in a 1950 monograph supplement to *Acta Otolaryngologica,* prepared by the clinic's first chief audiologist, Moe Bergman (Figure 4–2). In 1948 audiology clinics were opened in Washington, DC and Philadelphia.

Throughout the 1960s and 1970s, the VA sponsored summer training programs for audiology graduate students. Each student rotated through three VA clinics, gaining a unique perspective on the broad spectrum of audiologic services provided by the VA. Many of the participants of these summer programs went on to become leading clinicians and researchers, both in the VA and in other university and hospital settings.

It might be said, however, that the VA hearing aid program is the crown jewel of the enterprise. Beginning in the late 1950s, VA centers adapted the techniques developed in the earlier military programs to the needs of veterans. They put into place a procurement program that ensured quality

instruments, developed evaluation and treatment methods, refined electroacoustic evaluation of aids, and dispensed, to the veteran, the same aid with which he or she had been tested. And all this was happening while audiologists outside the VA and the military had to send candidates off to a hearing aid dealer for dispensation of an aid. Today, the VA continues to be the largest purchaser of hearing aids in the United States. One in every seven hearing aids dispensed in the United States is fitted by a VA audiologist.

Research has always been encouraged and funded within the VA system, and many significant contributions to the field have been made by VA audiologists. In 1997 the VA expanded its research program significantly by establishing the National Center for Rehabilitative Auditory Research (NCRAR) at the Portland VA Medical Center in Portland, Oregon. Under the direction of Stephen Fausti (Figure 4–3), the Center focuses entirely on audiologic research, the training of new audiological scientists, and dissemination

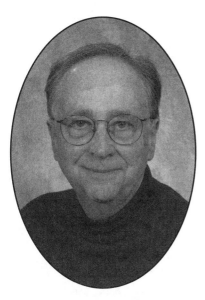

Figure 4-3. Stephen Fausti.

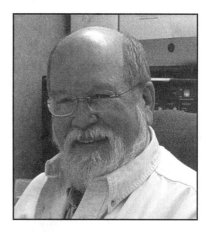

Figure 4-4. Richard Wilson. (Courtesy of the Department of Veterans Affairs.)

of research findings to clinicians who treat both veterans and nonveterans with hearing impairment. An important mission of the Center is to educate the general public about hearing conservation, how to prevent future loss, and how to cope with tinnitus.

Few people realize the extent to which the VA has supported the preparation of recorded speech audiometric materials. In the early 1950s, the VA and the Navy jointly funded the development of the recorded W-1, W-2, and W-22 disks by Ira Hirsh and his staff at the Central Institute for the Deaf. These recordings of spondee words (W-1 and W-2) and PB words (W-22) were, for many years, the only recorded materials available for speech audiometry. Over the past two decades Richard Wilson (Figure 4-4), chief of the audiology clinic at the Mountain Home, Tennessee VA facility, has collected almost all of the speech audiometric materials developed since the original W-1, W-2, and W-22 tests and has recorded them on compact disks for use within the VA system. In addition, the VA has generously made these disks available to the profession at large.

The VA system is now the largest employer of audiologists in the United States. Today, the VA employs 585 audiologists at 220 care sites. In a single year, 2004, VA audiologists treated more than 420,000 patients during more than 815,000 patient visits.

SECTION II

Six Divergent Paths

Over the six decades that have elapsed since the end of World War II audiology has evolved along six distinct and major paths: (1) a diagnostic path, emphasizing the use of auditory tests to sharpen the description and diagnosis of hearing disorders; (2) a rehabilitative path, underscoring procedures to counteract the effects of hearing disorders; (3) a pediatric path, emphasizing the early detection and assessment of hearing disorders; (4) an auditory processing disorder (APD) path stressing the evaluation and treatment of children and adults who seemed to have listening problems in spite of apparently normal peripheral auditory sensitivity; (5) a hearing conservation path; and (6) a tinnitus evaluation and therapy path. In the following chapters I have attempted to trace the major developments in each of these paths over the last half century.

5

Diagnosis

The Alternate Binaural Loudness Balance (ABLB)Test

One of the earliest diagnostic test procedures over and above the conventional tests for air and bone conduction threshold sensitivity was the alternate binaural loudness balance test (ABLB). Edmund Prince Fowler, an otolaryngologist at Columbia University, devised and developed this test in the late 1920s and 1930s as a procedure for comparing suprathreshold loudness at the two ears. It often revealed that, in spite of unilateral threshold hearing loss, loudness in the bad ear was achieved by suprathreshold sounds at the same intensity in the two ears, a phenomenon that came to be called "loudness recruitment." Fowler used the ABLB procedure to explore patients with unilateral otosclerosis, but did not learn very much that was useful. Later, however, the technique was used to great advantage in differentiating Ménière's disease from acoustic tumor.

One might view 1948 as the birth of site-of-lesion testing. In England, Dix, Hallpike, and Hood published a paper in the *Proceedings of the Royal Society of Medicine* in which they showed that one could differentiate between unilateral loss due to Ménière's disease from unilateral loss due to acoustic tumor, or to middle ear disorder, by means of Fowler's ABLB test. Patients with Ménière's disease showed partial or complete loudness recruitment, especially for high frequencies, but patients with conductive loss or with acoustic tumor did not. Figure 5–1, taken from Figure 2 of their paper, compares audiograms and ABLB findings in a case of unilateral conductive loss and a case of unilateral sensory neural loss ("nerve deafness"). In the case of the conductive loss (and in cases of acoustic tumor), the "laddergram" joining intensities judged equally loud on the two ears, shows parallel lines at all suprathreshold levels. But in the case of sensory neural loss, presumably localized in the cochlea, the laddergram shows that, in spite of the ear difference at threshold, by the time the hearing level is 80 dB in the poorer ear, it is judged as loud as the same intensity on the better ear. This convergence of lines on the laddergram was thought to be a direct measure of the loudness recruitment phenomenon, which could be used to differentiate unilateral disorders in the cochlea, like Ménière's disease, from unilateral disorders like acoustic tumor. Note that, on the audiograms, the right ear is denoted by an X and the left ear by a filled circle, exactly opposite to the convention used in the United States This 1948 publication by Dix, Hallpike, and Hood stirred a good deal of interest in the loudness recruitment phenomenon as a means of differentiating cochlear from retrocochlear site of disorder.

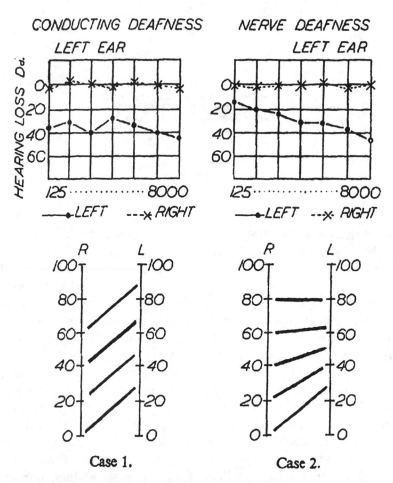

Figure 5–1. Laddergrams from the original publication of Dix, Hallpike, and Hood, in 1948, illustrating how the Alternate Binaural Loudness Balance (ABLB) test could be used to differentiate, on the one hand conductive and retrocochlear sites of disorder (*left side of figure*) from, on the other hand, inner ear sites (*right side of figure*). Two sources of confusion for current readers in the United States are the use of the term "nerve deafness" to refer to what we would now call a cochlear site, and the use of the symbols "O" for the left ear and "X" for the right ear. (Reprinted from the *Proceedings of the Royal Society of Medicine,* 1948, Fig. 2, on p. 517). Reproduced by permission of The Royal Society of Medicine, London.

The Intensity Difference Limen

The principal problem with ABLB as a clinical test was the fact that it could only be used effectively in patients with unilateral loss. How, people asked, can we detect loudness recruitment in patients with bilateral losses? Is there another way of getting at the apparent abnormal growth of loudness? In Switzerland, Professor E. Lüscher reasoned that, if loudness was growing too rapidly with intensity, then the difference limen for loudness, the smallest detectable loudness, must be smaller than in a normal ear. Could one then detect this by measuring the intensity DL at suprathreshold levels? He enlisted the aid of a young assistant with a background in electrical engineering, a Polish immigrant to Switzerland named Jozef Zwislocki (Figure 5–2). At the age of 17, Zwislocki had fled Poland in 1939 as the Germans invaded. He made his way to Switzerland and completed studies in electrical engineering in Basel, then took a job as lab assistant to Professor Lüscher. Together they crafted a device to measure the smallest detectable sinusoidal modulation in the amplitude of a continuous pure tone. They then applied it to patients in Lüscher's ENT clinic. Most patients with sensorineural loss did, indeed, show amplitude modulation thresholds well below the values characterizing normal ears at comparable sensation levels. Lüscher and Zwislocki suggested this as an "indirect" measure of the loudness recruitment phenomenon. Their findings created worldwide interest in how one might detect the presence of loudness recruitment "indirectly" and thereby facilitate the distinction between sensory and neural lesions of the auditory system.

In 1958, Carhart and Jerger published results on what later came to be called tone decay or abnormal adaptation. In 1953 and 1954, Jerger was running subjects for his dissertation research on intensity discrimination using the quantal psychophysical method. He presented a continuous tone at SL = 20 dB upon which were superimposed intensity increments to which the participant responded. Jerger recruited Ray Carhart as a subject for the experiment because Carhart had a deep notch at 4000 Hz due to an aspirin regimen he was undergoing. After the session, Carhart reported that, although he continued to hear the increments, the continuous carrier tone promptly faded away entirely. After a few minutes into the trial he couldn't hear it at all. Carhart and Jerger pursued this interesting observation with some acoustic tumor patients and found that they showed the same phenomenon to a remarkable degree. These findings led to the various tone decay and reflex decay tests that are still in use today.

Based on his work with short intensity increments, Jerger modified the classical quantal psychophysical method down to the presentation of 20 increments of exactly 1 dB at SL = 20 dB and called it the short-increment sensitivity index or SISI test. The bottom line was that patients with cochlear lesions could detect the increments with ease, especially at high frequencies, but patients with eighth nerve problems, or with conductive loss, could not. It was one of several tests that worked moderately well until supplanted by the auditory brainstem response (ABR).

Békésy Audiometry

The automatic audiometer was invented by Georg von Békésy during his time in Stockholm after he fled Hungary before World War II. But it received little clinical attention

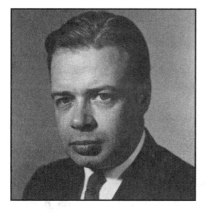

Figure 5–2. Jozef Zwislocki.

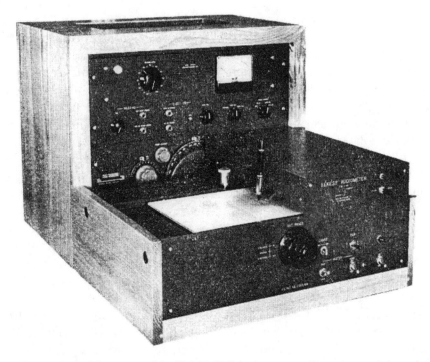

Figure 5–3. The venerable E-800 Békèsy-type audiometer, produced by the Grason-Stadler Company in the late 1950s and 1960s. From its use emerged the five types of Békèsy audiogram types, based on the difference between thresholds for continuous and temporally interrupted pure-tone stimuli. Reprinted with permission from Jerger, J. (1963). *Modern Developments in Audiology.* New York: Academic Press (Fig. 3, p. 40).

until the late 1950s when the Grason-Stadler Company produced a commercial instrument, the venerable E-800 (Figure 5–3). At Northwestern, Jerger bought one of the first units and ran some 400 patients through the procedure. In Békésy's original instrument, the test tone was on continuously, but on the E-800 there was the option of periodically interrupting the continuous test tone. Based on an earlier suggestion by Peter Denes, Jerger thought it might be useful to test in both the continuous and interrupted modes. This turned up the four Békésy types; type I in normals and conductive disorders, type II in cochlear disorders, and types III and IV in VIIIth nerve disorders. Later, Gilbert Herer

added a type V, in which the continuous trace runs well above the interrupted trace, a sign of functional and malingering losses (pseudohypacusis).

Pseudohypacusis

Pseudohypacusis, itself, has had an interesting history. The earliest reported case is unknown, but by the end of World War I there were many anecdotal reports of military personnel who consciously feigned hearing loss to avoid hazardous assignments. Early attempts to unmask such individuals were primitive at best (e.g., standing behind the suspect and telling an assistant, at a normal vocal level, that the suspect's fly was unzipped). But by the end of World War II, more formal techniques had been worked out. They included the Lombard test, the Doerfler-Stewart test, the Swinging Voice test, the Stenger test, and, in the case of feigned unilateral loss, the absence of an appropriate "shadow curve." As service-connected losses were subject to monetary compensation, the Veterans Administration devoted substantial resources to the development of reliable techniques for detecting pseudohypacusis.

In the civilian sector, pseudohypacusis became a problem in industries where workers were exposed to high levels of noise for extended periods. As genuine losses from such environmental stress became monetarily compensable, it was inevitable that some workers would feign loss to receive such compensation. But here the problem was compounded by the fact that a pseudohypacusic loss might overlay a genuine loss resulting from the extended noise exposure. And, as Maurice Miller (Figure 5–4) and his colleagues at New York University have argued, a pseudohypacusic loss may overlay a life-threatening retrocochlear disorder.

The search for better methods of unmasking and quantifying the pseudohypacusic component was greatly facilitated by the advent of the auditory brainstem response, the N1-P2 complex, and otoacoustic emissions.

Dichotic Tests

The dichotic listening paradigm has become a powerful tool for the study of linguistic processing. It is used to great advantage by psychologists, neurophysiologists, audiologists, and a number of other disciplines. The procedure was originally devised by a British psychologist, Donald Broadbent, who marveled at the ability of air traffic controllers to seemingly monitor several ongoing events simultaneously. To study the phenomenon in the laboratory, he devised a technique in which one or more pairs of digits are heard simultaneously in the two ears. The listener must report what was heard in any order. The modern Dichotic Digits test derives from this early work.

In 1961 Brenda Milner and Doreen Kimura, of the Montreal Neurological Institute applied Broadbent's dichotic paradigm to the study of patients with brain disorders. This was a good example of the fact that you don't always need sophisticated equipment to make fundamental discoveries. Milner and Kimura had recorded the digit stimuli on what one can only charitably describe as a low-end tape recorder, the sort that speech clinicians like to use to record faulty patient utterances. But with this simple instrumentation they discovered the right-ear advantage in dichotic listening and spawned an area of research on hemispheric asymmetry and hemispheric specialization that continues

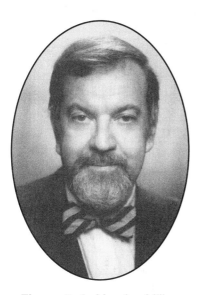

Figure 5–4. Maurice Miller.

to pay dividends to this day. Doreen Kimura published the seminal findings in the *Canadian Journal of Psychology* in 1961.

Impedance (Immittance) Audiometry

In 1946 Otto Metz of Denmark developed the first viable middle-ear impedance bridge. Metz built a fairly unwieldy gadget, principally to detect contraction of the middle-ear muscles. Figure 5–5 illustrates the principle. A diaphragm driven by an oscillator was mounted between two fairly long tubes. One tube was sealed in the ear canal, the other terminated in a device permitting variation in the volume of the tube. The tone in one tube was, of course, 180 degrees out of phase with the tone in the other tube. The operator, listening through a stethoscope, adjusted the volume, or "compliance," of the far tube until a null was heard in the tones in the tubes. Then a loud tone was introduced to the opposite ear via an audiometer. If the stapedius muscle contracted, the "bridge" became unbalanced, due to the increase in the stiffness of the middle ear mechanical system caused by the muscle contraction and the

null was lost. By varying the intensity of the stimulating tone, one could, in this fashion, determine the "acoustic reflex threshold." Using the device, Metz was able to demonstrate loudness recruitment as a reduction in the sensation level of the tone eliciting a reflex contraction of the stapedius muscle.

In 1963 Jozef Zwislocki attempted to improve on the Otto Metz impedance bridge by adding a way to measure both absolute resistance and reactance (compliance), and by making everything much smaller (Figure 5–6). The only problem was that it took a three-handed person to carry this out. You needed one hand to hold the instrument in the ear canal, a second hand to move the compliance plunger in and out, and a third hand to turn the resistance adjuster. The device never really caught on clinically, but it served the important function of arousing great interest in the possibilities of impedance audiometry (later called "immittance audiometry") in the United States. Zwislocki founded the Institute for Sensory Research at Syracuse University and has made seminal contributions to many areas of hearing science, especially auditory psychophysics and biophysics, throughout his distinguished research career.

The Metz Device

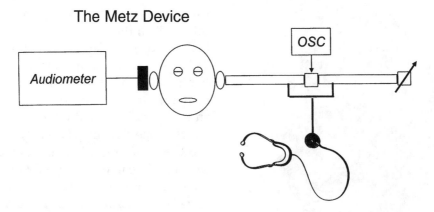

Figure 5–5. One of the earliest impedance bridges, designed by Otto Metz of Denmark. It was used to detect contractions of the stapedius muscle (the aural reflex) when an intense sound was presented to the opposite ear.

The Zwislocki Bridge

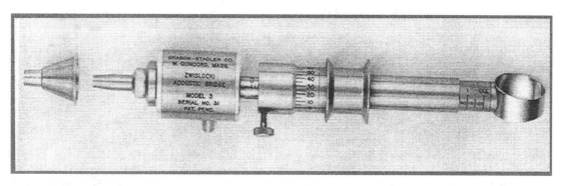

Figure 5–6. The Zwislocki impedance bridge introduced in the early 1960s. It permitted the measurement of the absolute impedance characteristics of the middle ear mechanism, but was difficult to use clinically. (Reprinted from *Acoustic Impedance and Admittance*, Williams and Wilkins, 1976.)

What we now know as tympanometry was pioneered by Gunnar Lidén in Sweden. His 1969 paper, in the *Journal of Laryngology and Otology*, laid out the basis for the relation between middle-ear pathology and tympanometric morphology. The first paper on tympanometry in the United States, based on the collaboration of Lidén and Earl Harford at Northwestern University, was presented by Harford at the ASHA convention in Denver in 1968.

The clinical exploitation of immittance audiometry, however, awaited the development of an electroacoustic measuring device. In 1970 the first really usable instruments for measuring middle ear impedance characteristics and acoustic reflex measurement were produced by the Madsen company in Denmark, the ZO-70 impedance bridge (Figure 5–7).

Jerger was at the Baylor College of Medicine in Houston at the time and managed to acquire one of the earliest of the ZO-70 instruments. Following Bunch's example, he simply had his audiologists run every patient through the procedure. After some 400 cases had been tested, the clinical value of impedance testing became evident. Absolute impedance measures, which had been the driving force behind the development of these instruments, turned out to be the least interesting data. The real value was in exploring tympanograms and the stapedius muscle reflex. Jerger's 1970 publication on all of this, in the *AMA Archives of Otolaryngology*, continues to be a frequently cited reference 35 years later. Within the last two decades, many individuals have advanced the science of middle-ear measurement beyond the earliest applications; particularly noteworthy has been the work of Robert Margolis (Figure 5–8) of the University of Minnesota.

Auditory Evoked Potentials

Nineteen thirty-nine (1939) saw the first description of alteration in brain waves due to auditory stimulation. A young physiologist at Harvard University, Pauline Davis, first wife of Hallowell Davis, observed perturbations

The Madsen Bridge

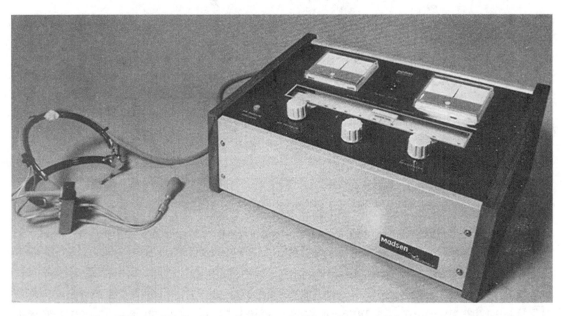

Figure 5–7. The ZO-70 Madsen electroacoustic impedance bridge, introduced in the late 1960s. Its comparative ease of use fueled clinical interest in what has come to be called "immittance audiometry."

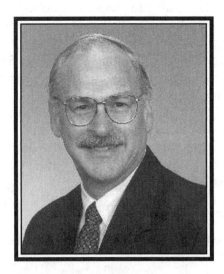

Figure 5–8. Robert Margolis.

"K-complex." Unfortunately, this was some years before the advent of averaging computers, and the finding could not be immediately exploited.

Historically, the first averaged auditory evoked potential to be described was what we now call the middle latency response or MLR. In 1958 Dan Geisler (Figure 5–9), then at the University of Chicago, using an early digital computer, noted a consistent positivity in the latency region of 30 to 40 msec, which we now call Pa. Historically this was the first in the family of auditory evoked potentials to be described. It was later studied at great length by Robert Goldstein and his students, first at Jewish Hospital in St. Louis, and later at the University of Wisconsin-Madison.

What is now known as the N1-P2 complex, in the 100- to 250-msec latency range, was the second auditory evoked potential to be identified. Hallowell Davis, working

in ongoing alpha activity recorded from scalp electrodes when sounds were presented to the ear. The Davises named it the

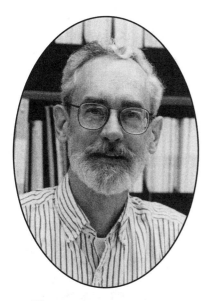

Figure 5–9. Dan Geisler.

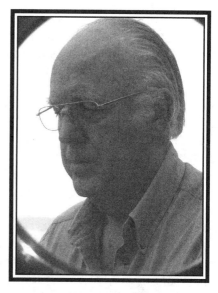

Figure 5–10. Donald Jewett.

at the Central Institute for the Deaf, called it the "vertex potential" because it was largest at the CZ or vertex electrode. Davis and his colleagues spent a good deal of time in the 1960s vainly attempting to exploit the vertex potential as a test of hearing in infants and other difficult-to-test children. But it never really worked too well, largely because of the labile state of the young brain. In recent years, this response has been used successfully in auditory perceptual studies and in the evaluation of children and adults with cochlear implants.

Few test procedures have had the same profound effect on audiologic practice as the third evoked potential discovered, the auditory brainstem response (ABR). It has truly revolutionized diagnostic evaluation. Gone are SISI, ABLB, and Békésy-type audiograms. They have been replaced by a single powerful tool that differentiates cochlear from VIIIth nerve sites with high sensitivity and acceptable specificity, a tool that has made it possible to detect hearing loss in children virtually from birth. In the early 1970s, Donald Jewett (Figure 5–10), then a postdoctoral fellow in the laboratory of Robert Galambos at Yale University, stumbled upon this response almost by accident. He was studying later evoked responses in the cat when he noticed what appeared to be four repeatable bumps in the first 10 msec after stimulus onset. Later, as a faculty member at the University of California at San Francisco (UCSF), Jewett found five repeatable bumps in the same latency region in humans. Previous investigators had missed them because it was the fashion in those days to band-pass filter the EEG rather narrowly around the frequency region of interest, which for the middle and late responses was well below 100 Hz. Thus, EEG activity in the 500- to 1000-Hz range, where the ABR response is maximal, was, in effect, discarded. But Jewett wisely avoided such narrow filtering and made an historic discovery. It turned out that the second wave of the human ABR was equivalent to the first wave of the cat ABR. To avoid confusion, Jewett used arabic numerals for the four peaks of the cat ABR and roman numerals for the five peaks of the human ABR.

Clearly, the ABR has had a tremendous effect on diagnostic evaluation in our field. For the audiology student, the wealth of research on various aspects of the ABR has been effectively collected into a single volume by Jay Hall III (Figure 5–11), of the University of Florida.

Within the past decade, Nina Kraus (Figure 5–12) and colleagues at Northwestern University have shown that the ABR response to speech and music sounds reflects the timing, harmonic, and pitch elements of key events of the speech or music waveform. Results have profoundly influenced our understanding of the neural correlates of auditory training and have been unusually useful in evaluating the auditory perceptual problems encountered in some language-impaired children who experience difficulty reading and listening in noise.

The late Sam Sutton, of the New York State Psychiatric Institute, is credited with the first description of a cognitive potential evoked by the occurrence of a rare or unique event. Early investigations of the phenomenon studied the response to a relatively rarely occurring 2000-Hz tone burst randomly interspersed among more frequent 1000 Hz tone bursts (that is, the "oddball" paradigm). As in this paradigm, the evoked response to the rare event was characterized by a positivity in the latency region of 300 msec, it was originally called the P300. Subsequent investigators have shown, however, that the response can be evoked over a wide range of latencies depending on the nature and difficulty of the task. It is now called an event-related potential, or ERP, and the unique positivity, thought to be related to an updating of working memory, is called the late positive component, or LPC. The ERP is exceedingly flexible and has many applications in audiologic evaluation. The LPC occurs in the latency region of 300

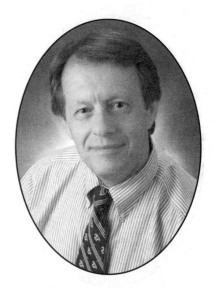

Figure 5–11. Jay Hall III.

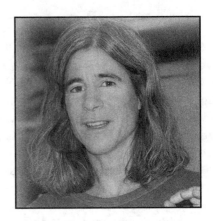

Figure 5–12. Nina Kraus.

to 900 msec. In the three decades since the first description of this cognitive potential, a number of other ERPs have been discovered, including the N2, a negativity at about 220 msec, thought to index phonological processing; the mismatch negativity response (MMN), thought to reflect acoustic analysis of the stimulus; the N400, negativity in the 400-msec latency range, reflecting semantic processing, especially semantic incongruity; the P600, a positivity in the 500- to 700-msec range, indexing syntactic incongruity, and the auditory steady state response (ASSR) which is proving to be valuable in the testing of young children.

Among the studies of the many individuals in this country actively pursuing ASSR research in the pediatric population, the work of Barbara Cone-Wesson (Figure 5–13), at the University of Arizona, has been particularly noteworthy. Recently, Jennifer Shinn and Frank Musiek have suggested another possible application of ASSR, assisting in the detection of neurologic insult of the central auditory nervous system.

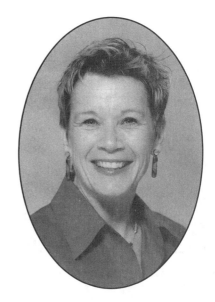

Figure 5–13. Barbara Cone-Wesson.

Otoacoustic Emissions

The successful recording of evoked and spontaneous emissions from the inner ear, by David Kemp (Figure 5–14), in 1978, set off a flurry of activity around the world. It seemed that here, at last, we might have a truly objective method for measuring degree of hearing sensitivity loss without the need for active cooperation from the person being evaluated. As luck would have it, the measure turned out to be too sensitive. It is so sensitive to the status of the outer hair cells that it drops out altogether when degree of loss exceeds 40 to 50 dB. But, as so often happens in our field, other applications of otoacoustic emissions (OAEs) have turned out to be even more interesting and valuable.

Of the many researchers who have contributed to the basic science of otoacoustic emissions, and to their clinical applications, we may single out for particular note Michael Gorga and his colleagues, at the Boys Town Institute, Brenda Lonsbury-Martin and Glen Martin of Loma Linda University, Martin Robinette of the Mayo Clinics, Yvonne Sin-

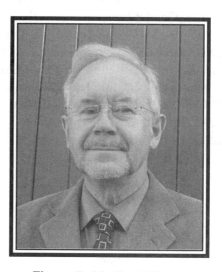

Figure 5–14. David Kemp.

inger of UCLA, and Ted Glattke of the University of Arizona.

One such application, the efferent suppression of OAEs, first described by Lionel Collet and his colleagues in France, continues to show great promise in the evaluation of central auditory processing, especially at the

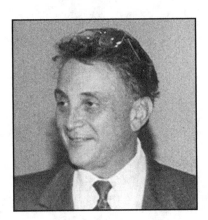

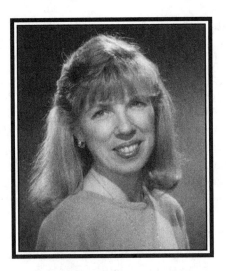

Figure 5–15. Charles Berlin. (Courtesy of Harriet Berlin.)

Figure 5–16. Linda Hood.

low brainstem level. Ever at the forefront of innovation, Charles Berlin (Figure 5–15), Linda Hood (Figure 5–16), and their colleagues at the LSU Medical Center pioneered the clinical applications of efferent suppression. Their work will certainly lead to significant breakthroughs in our understanding of the complex interactions among afferent and efferent effects in the auditory system.

Sensitized Tests

In the early 1950s, a group of investigators in Italy led by Ettore Bocca, approached the study of central auditory processing problems by testing neurologic patients with temporal lobe disorders. These investigators, especially A. R. Antonelli and G. P. Teatini, showed that, although such patients had no difficulty understanding simple speech in either ear, when the listening task was made more difficult, either by low-pass filtering or temporal speeding, performance on the ear contralateral to the affected side of the brain was noticeably poorer than performance on the ipsilateral ear. They called their measures "sensitized speech audiometry." The findings stirred great interest, especially among American investigators seeking a better understanding of the effects of brain lesions on auditory perception. Many of our current tests for auditory processing disorder derive from this early work by the pioneering Italians.

Frank Musiek (Figure 5–17), of the University of Connecticut, has been a tireless worker in the development and evaluation of a wide variety of tests for auditory function in the neurologically impaired. Together with his colleagues, Jane Baran and Marilyn Pinheiro, he has developed tests of frequency and duration pattern ability, tests of gap detection, and has exploited a variety of dichotic procedures, as well as the full range of auditory evoked responses, in his studies of brain-injured individuals. Musiek coined the term "neuroaudiology" to highlight this unique application of audiologic expertise, and has written extensively in the area.

As early as 1948, John Gaeth (Figure 5–18), after studying word recognition in an elderly cohort, concluded that one could not fully explain all of their word recognition

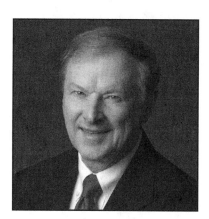

Figure 5–17. Frank Musiek.

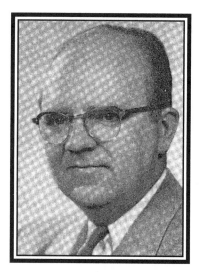

Figure 5–18. John Gaeth.

scores from the audiogram alone. Something else seemed to be reducing PB max scores in some elderly individuals. He named the phenomenon "phonemic regression." Five decades later, many still find this concept difficult to accept but we now know that, in addition to the undeniably important audibility factor, there are age-related changes in frequency resolution, temporal resolution, cognition, and central auditory processing.

Many audiologists have contributed importantly to a comparative evaluation of the various diagnostic procedures that have been proposed over the years. Particularly insightful were the comprehensive studies of patient groups by Douglas Noffsinger and Wayne Olsen (Figure 5–19), then at Northwestern University. Their work paved the way for a much needed winnowing of techniques to ensure maximal efficiency in diagnostic evaluation.

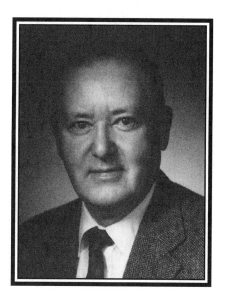

Figure 5–19. Wayne Olsen.

6

Rehabilitation

Throughout much of the history of modern audiology the principal rehabilitative weapons have been wearable hearing aids, assistive devices, cochlear implants, and auditory training. Their paths have become interestingly intertwined.

Hearing Aids

Leland Watson, president of the Maico Company, and Thomas Tolan, an otolaryngologist, traced, in their volume, *Hearing Tests and Hearing Instruments*, the early history of the development of the wearable hearing aid. The following is based on their comprehensive review.

Alexander Graham Bell played a significant role in the invention of the first electrical hearing aid. In an effort to help his hearing-impaired wife, he experimented with the electrical properties of carbon granules. Bell failed to succeed with the hearing aid project, but his work with carbon granules led directly to the invention of the telephone. The first viable hearing aid based on carbon granule technology was actually developed by a Viennese physician, Dr. Ferdinand Alt, in 1900. American versions were produced in 1902 by Miller Reese Hutchinson in Mobile, Alabama and C. W. Harper in Boston. Carbon-granule based hearing aids were widely available in the 1920s and 1930s, but they had many problems, not the least of which was fairly poor sound quality. Vacuum tube amplifiers were a giant step forward. The first vacuum tube-based aid in the United States was produced by Art Wengel in 1937. It was called the "Stanleyphone." But it remained for the Aurex company to make the technology widely available. These aids stretched the definition of portable to an extreme degree. They were powered by a separate battery pack. The amplifying unit was mounted somewhere on the upper body, the battery pack either strapped to the midsection or on one leg. How a contemporary woman might outfit herself in the 1930s is illustrated in Figure 6–1.

The truly wearable hearing aid was made possible by the invention, and systematic improvement, of the miniature vacuum tube in the late 1930s. The filaments of the tubes were heated by a 1.5-volt "A" battery, the plate biased by a 22- to 30-volt "B" battery. These aids, about the size of a package of cigarettes, could be worn in a shirt pocket or in a cloth pocket suspended from the neck. They were connected by thin wire to a small transducer, curiously referred to as a "receiver," mounted in the ear canal by a totally occluding earmold. Such aids were made available to the aural rehabilitative

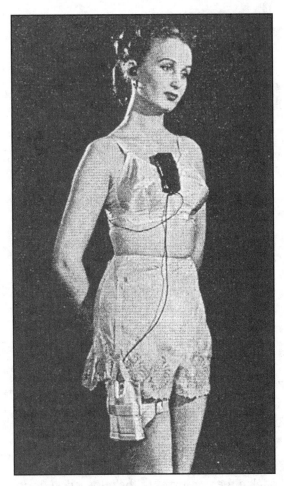

Figure 6–1. How a hearing aid was worn in the 1930s. The amplifying unit, mounted on the chest, was supplied by batteries strapped to one leg, and was connected by a long, flexible wire to the transducer mounted in a fully occluding earmold. (Reprinted from *Hearing and Deafness*, first edition, Murray Hill Books, 1947.)

programs of the various services during and after World War II and were widely distributed to returning servicemen. Examples of these "all-in-one" aids are shown in Figure 6–2.

Sound quality, in these aids, was still marginal. Figure 6–3 shows the frequency response of one such aid at various tone con-

trol settings. The wide-band, flat response was still a few years away.

The military programs generated a long-standing debate, which at times became quite contentious, over what might be called the "philosophy of fitting" an aid. On the one hand were the exponents of "hearing aid selection," a procedure promoted most notably by Raymond Carhart and his many students. The rationale here was that the audiologist must seek, through objective testing of speech understanding, the aid that best matches the unique shape and degree of the serviceman's loss. This was achieved by manipulation of gain and tone control of each of several candidate aids in search of optimal word intelligibility. As outcome measures of this approach Carhart adapted, for this purpose, the speech audiometric scores based on the spondee and PB word lists developed at the Harvard Psychoacoustic Laboratory during the war. The underlying assumption of the hearing aid selection procedure was that individuals differed in the unique details of their losses and that the best aid was the aid that complemented the shape of the loss, especially in terms of its frequency response. It was assumed that the speech audiometric scores would order the aids appropriately.

As early as 1946, however, an alternative philosophy emerged from two sources: (1) the British Medical Research Council (MEDRESCO) hearing aid, and (2) the Harvard Report. The MEDRESCO aid was developed by British engineers to meet the needs of the nascent British National Health Service. They were convinced that a single, relatively flat, frequency response was sufficient for most hearing-impaired individuals. Thus, they allowed for only minimal adjustment of the tone control of the aid.

The Harvard Report was generated by a group of scientists, including as noted earlier, Hallowell Davis, working on the National

1948

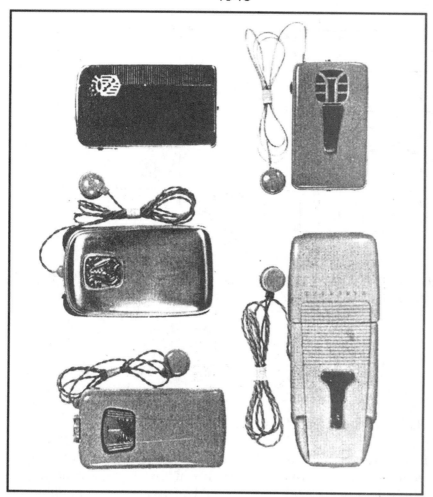

1998

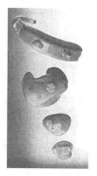

Figure 6–2. Five hearing aids popular in 1948, compared with four hearing aids popular in 1998. Fifty years of miniaturization.

Defense Research Council (NDRC) Aural Rehabilitation Project at Harvard University during the last years of World War II. They tested a number of hearing-impaired individuals with a master hearing aid, in which the frequency response could be manipulated over a wide range. Their report, published in 1946, reinforced the MEDRESCO philosophy in concluding that selective amplification was of little value. A uniform (flat) frequency response, or a response slightly tilted upward in the high frequencies, almost always yielded the best speech understanding scores. Thus, elaborate selection procedures were not warranted. For the next several decades, lively debate ensued between proponents of the two conflicting philosophies. Traditionalists continued to carry out hearing aid selection testing in the Carhart manner while young turks called for reform, but usually to little avail. It must be said, however, that the physical characteristics of the aids of that era

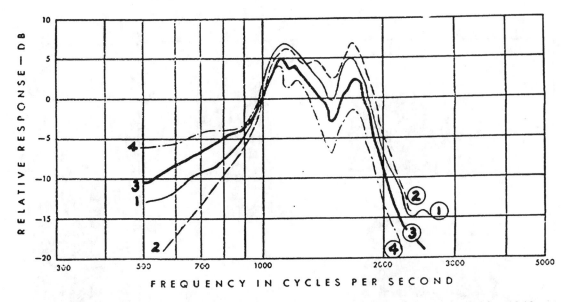

Figure 6–3. The frequency response of an inexpensive hearing aid popular in the 1940s at four positions of the tone control. (Reprinted from *Hearing Tests and Hearing Instruments*, Williams & Wilkins, 1949.)

did not permit very precise control over the frequency response of any aid. In retrospect, it is doubtful that either side could have amassed very much hard evidence in support of its position.

A similar conclusion was reached as early as 1949 by none other than Harvey Fletcher himself. He opined, at the Second Congress of the International Society of Audiology, that the appropriate frequency response of an aid ought to simply mirror the audiometric threshold levels, but that there would be little difference in word recognition scores between such an aid and one with a flat frequency response, so that, for all practical purposes the aid with a flat response should be suitable for everyone. He did concede, however, that if the audiogram sloped downward by more than 20 dB between 500 and 2000 Hz, then the response of the aid should slope upward at about one third the slope of the audiometric contour.

In the early 1950s the transistor was developed and its value in the design of wearable aids was immediately apparent. Transistors were certainly a good deal smaller than miniature vacuum tubes, but the main advantage was the elimination of the need for the bulky, high-voltage "B" battery. Transistors could manage the same amplification powered only by a small 1.5-volt "A" battery. This additional miniaturization made it possible to move the amplifier unit from the chest to a location over and behind the auricle, the behind-the-ear unit, and ultimately into the ear canal itself. Miniaturization also made bilateral fittings feasible, permitting for the first time the capability of exploiting the several advantages of two-eared hearing.

One of the early attempts in this direction was the development of the "eyeglass aid" in the 1960s. In this novel arrangement all of the components of an aid were built into the eyeglass frames, one aid on each side. It was a clever idea, but never really caught on, perhaps because it complicated the process of taking the glasses off and putting them back on. In those days, heavy frames were in vogue, but as that fad passed away, and only thin wire frames remained, there was no longer space for the hearing aids and the era of the eyeglass aid passed away with little fanfare.

An interesting innovation in hearing aid configuration was suggested by Earl Harford (Figure 6–4) and Joseph Barry in 1965. Persons with severe or profound unilateral loss were not considered suitable for hearing aid fitting because of the normal or near normal hearing on the better ear. But these individuals frequently complained of difficulty when the talker was on the side of the poorer hearing ear and difficulty in telling the direction from which a sound was coming. Harford and Barry reasoned that such a person might be helped by a fitting in which the aid and its microphone were mounted on the poorer hearing ear but the signal was actually routed to the better hearing ear. They called this arrangement CROS, standing for "contralateral routing of signal." Several innovative arrangements of the CROS principle were subsequently devised, including FM transmission of the signal from one side of the head to the other. In 1966 Harford further suggested that an individual with loss in both ears, but substantially more loss in one ear than the other, might benefit from a BICROS arrangement in which two aids are fitted but both signals are routed to the better ear.

The development of real-ear measurement of hearing aid performance was pioneered by Earl Harford. In the early 1970s, the advent of the miniature Knowles microphone raised the possibility of actually recording the sound pressure level of a signal within the human ear canal. Up to this time, hearing aid performance typically had been measured on a 2-cc coupler. But this approach failed to take into account the variations in response due to differences in real ear canals, transducer placement, and so forth. In 1973, William (Bill) Austin and David Preves of Starkey Laboratories brought samples of the new microphone to Harford's lab at Northwestern University and the trio ran numerous tests, using themselves as subjects, of what we now know as real-ear-measurement techniques. Austin and Preves continued to provide even smaller Knowles mikes as Harford continued his work testing hundreds of patients at the University of Minnesota. The first paper on the subject was presented by Harford at an International Symposium on Sensorineural Hearing Loss in Minneapolis in 1979. His first published paper, entitled "The Use of a Probe Microphone in the Ear Canal for the Measurement of Hearing Aid Performance," appeared a year later in *Ear and Hearing*. By 1985 clinically useful real-ear measurement systems were widely commercially available. In the almost 30 years since the original publications, real-ear measurement of hearing aid performance has become an essential element in the fitting of aids.

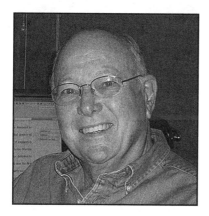

Figure 6–4. Earl Harford.

In addition to his seminal studies of bone conduction calibration and measurement, and his fundamental studies of speech recognition, the research of Donald Dirks (Figure 6–5), in particular, will be remembered for his development, with Sam Gilman, of a probe tube used to establish the effects of standing waves in the external ear canal over a wide range of frequencies. They were extremely useful in the subsequent development of clinical methods for real-ear measurement via probe microphones.

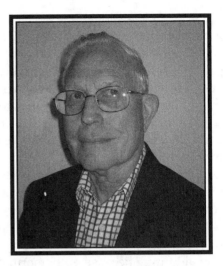

Figure 6–5. Donald Dirks. (Courtesy of Laraine Mestman.)

Auditory Deprivation and Acclimitization

In 1984 Shlomo Silman (Figure 6–6), Stanley Gelfand, and Carole Silverman published a seminal paper on auditory deprivation. When a person was aided monaurally, the aided ear maintained its speech-understanding capacity over time, whereas the unaided ear gradually declined. The late Stuart Gatehouse, in Scotland, later expanded the concept to include acclimatization, the tendency for the aided ear to improve slightly over time compared to the unaided ear. This important theoretical development has provided strong support for the fitting of aids to both ears whenever possible, even when there is a substantial difference between sensitivity levels on the two ears. It has also alerted researchers to take the initial period of acclimatization into account in hearing aid outcome research.

Binaural Aids

The fitting of independent bilateral aids, one to each ear, has had an interesting history.

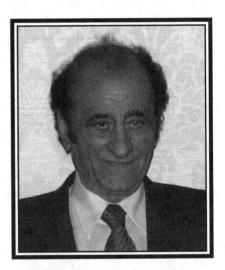

Figure 6–6. Shlomo Silman.

The idea that both ears ought to be aided in order to take advantage of the benefits of two-eared hearing was commonly asserted from the very earliest days of hearing aid fitting. But it was not until the advent of transistors that miniaturization made it practical to mount the aids, and their microphones in or near the two ears. Such fittings were originally called "binaural," but the late Dennis

Bryne of the National Acoustic Laboratory in Sydney, Australia suggested that a more appropriate term would be "bilateral" in recognition of the fact that bilateral aids do not necessarily restore normal binaural function.

In spite of accumulating research evidence that bilateral hearing was, on average, superior to unilateral hearing in persons with normal two-eared hearing, for many years, there was considerable resistance in the marketplace to the fitting of an aid to each ear, probably for two principal reasons: (1) the additional cost of the second aid was a deterrent for many potential users, and (2) conventional speech audiometric test materials seldom reflected, in hearing-impaired individuals, the two-eared advantage so well documented in persons with normal hearing. As this situation improved, with the development of more sensitive tests; however, another problem surfaced. As more and more bilateral aids were fit, especially to elderly persons, it became evident that not all individuals benefited from bilateral fittings to the same degree. Indeed, in some individuals, the presence of the second aid seemed to actually make matters worse. The problem was noted as early as 1939 by Vern Knudsen of UCLA, and by Leland Watson and Thomas Tolan. Watson and Tolan reported that their observations led them to suspect some kind of conflict between the two ears.

The phenomenon of binaural interference, described by Jerger and by Shlomo Silman in the 1980s and 1990s seemed to be at fault. In 2005 the problem was highlighted in a landmark study by Therese Walden and Brian Walden at the Walter Reed Army Medical Center. They showed that some elderly hearing aid users did, indeed, perform better on a test of speech understanding in competition when only one ear was aided. Performance was often poorest when both ears were aided. We still await data on the prevalence of this binaural interference phenomenon in the entire population of hearing-impaired individuals. It is certainly the case that the majority of hearing aid users of all ages perform better with a bilateral fitting, but the lesson for audiologists has been that all potential users, but especially elderly users, must be evaluated under both unilateral and bilateral fitting conditions.

Digital Signal Processing and Microphone Technology

No engineering advance in the past half century has had greater impact on the wearable hearing aid than the advent of digital signal processing in the late 1980s and early 1990s. Now, for the first time, it was possible to actually manipulate the fine grain of the frequency response of an aid in order to match it to the shape of the audiometric contour. This capability, combined with digital compression/expansion and various adaptive algorithms fueled a resurgence in interest in selective amplification. At the same time, studies by David Pascoe and Margo Skinner, at Washington University in St. Louis, by Larry Humes (Figure 6–7) at Indiana University, and by many other investigators, have emphasized the critical impact of the exact degree and configuration of high-frequency sensitivity loss on speech understanding. These two forces have lent such strong support to the philosophy of selective amplification that it has become the virtual rule in hearing aid fitting. Additionally, the laborious testing characterizing Carhart's original concept of hearing aid evaluation have given way to emphasis on fine tuning a smaller number of aids, with heavy reliance on the real-ear measurement of their physical characteristics.

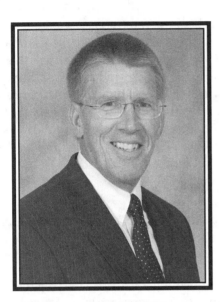

Figure 6–7. Larry Humes. (Courtesy of Indiana University Photo Services.)

Confluent with advances in digital signal processing, microphone technology has advanced to a point permitting the development of a truly directional microphone in which directivity patterns favoring input from a particular direction have been implemented. Although there have been voices of dissent, the available evidence seems to favor the use of directional microphones in most listening situations involving competing speech or noise.

In the months and years to come, it is certain that continuing advances in hearing aid technology will broaden our rehabilitative capabilities. Indeed, we are already seeing aids that learn a client's preferred volume setting, and switch among programs for quiet listening, music, listening to speech alone, and listening to speech in a noisy background. And there are aids that will automatically switch to the directional mode when background noise is detected, aids that can be recharged, and even aids that can be individually programmed to suit a particular lifestyle.

Accountability

As hearing aids and other amplification devices have become more sophisticated, there has been a growing sense that the field stands in need of better outcome measures to assess how well a particular intervention actually helps the hearing-impaired person. For many years, the only outcome measure available was the ubiquitous aided PB score. But Harvey Fletcher's prediction in 1949, that existing word recognition tests were not really capable of differentiating among aids, became ever more evident.

The efficacy of word discrimination testing, as it was then called, was challenged as early as 1960 by Irvin Shore, Robert Bilger, and Ira Hirsh at Central Institute for the Deaf. For the next two decades, there was growing unease about whether PB scores were acceptable as measures of accountability. Finally, in 1983, a study by Brian Walden and his colleagues at Walter Reed reinforced the growing feeling that word discrimination scores were just not up to the task.

Further development took three directions. First, there was a concerted effort to design more sophisticated measures of speech understanding such as the speech perception–in-noise (SPIN) test by Kalikow, Stevens, and Elliott in 1977 and its revised version by Bilger, Nuetzel, Rabinowitz, and Rzeczkowski in 1984, the hearing-in-noise test (HINT) by Nilson, Soli, and Sullivan in 1994, the BKB-speech-in-noise (BKB-SIN) test by Killion et al. in 1997, and its abbreviated version, the QUICKSin test in 2004. New tests will eventually replace the old PB lists, but progress is painfully slow.

A second major development has been the construction of assessment questionnaires such as the Hearing Handicap Inventory for the Elderly (HHIE) by Ira Ventry and Barbara

Weinstein in 1982, the Abbreviated Profile of Hearing Aid Benefit (APHAB) by Robyn Cox and Genevieve Alexander in 1995, the Client-Oriented Scale of Improvement (COSI) by Harvey Dillon in 1997, the Satisfaction with Amplification in Daily Life (SADL) scale by Cox and Alexander in 1999, and the International Outcome Inventory for Hearing Aids (IOI-HA) by Cox and Alexander in 2002. Researcher Robyn Cox (Figure 6–8), at the Memphis Speech and Hearing Center at the University of Memphis, has been one of the foremost supporters of accountability through evidence-based practice in audiology. Craig Newman (Figure 6–9), of the Cleveland Clinic, has been particularly active in the construction and evaluation of questionnaires in a number of areas including hearing handicap in the elderly, tinnitus evaluation, and quantifying hearing aid benefit.

A third development has been the application of cost-benefit analysis to aural intervention by Harvey Abrams and his colleagues at the VA Medical Center in Bay Pines, Florida.

Finally, there is the intriguing development of the concept of acceptable noise level as a predictor of a successful fitting by Anna Nabelek (Figure 6–10) and her colleagues

and students at the University of Tennessee-Knoxville.

Many audiologists have made significant contributions to research on hearing aids over the years. Space limitations preclude an exhaustive list, but a sampling of entrants to

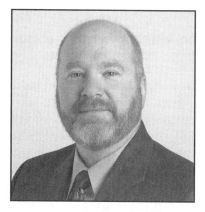

Figure 6–9. Craig Newman. (Courtesy of the Center for Medical Art and Photography, Cleveland Clinic.)

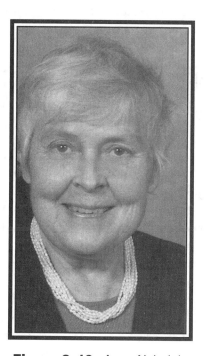

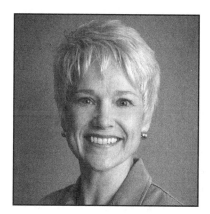

Figure 6–8. Robyn Cox. (University of Memphis, courtesy of L. Lissau.)

Figure 6–10. Anna Nabelek.

the hearing aid hall of fame would surely include Ruth Bentler, Donald Dirks, David Hawkins, Mead Killion, Sam Lybarger, David Pascoe, David Preves, Todd Ricketts, Margot Skinner, Wayne Staab, Pat Stelmachowicz, Gerald Studebaker, Tom Tillman, Michael Valente, and Laura Wilber.

The Saga of Barry Elpern

No history of audiologists and hearing aids would be complete without an account of the adventures and misadventures of Barry Elpern (Figure 6–11). Barry was an audiologist at the University of Chicago in the 1960s. One cold mid-winter evening in 1967, he was driving home from work on Chicago's south side in the midst of a record-setting midwestern blizzard. Snow and freezing wind swirled around his car as he made his way, slowly and stressfully, along the freeway. But it soon became impassable. After spending the night in his car, he had to walk

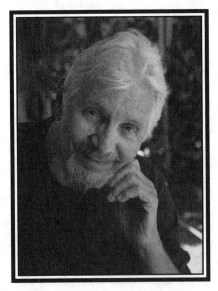

Figure 6–11. Barry Elpern.

the rest of the way home in cold, waist-deep snow. He describes a moment of epiphany, during this walk, in which he asked himself, "Is this any way for a reasonable person to live?" As soon as he reached home he instructed his family to pack up as they were moving to Arizona.

In Phoenix, Barry joined a group of engineers who had formed a company to improve hearing aid performance. As part of the operation, they established a dispensary to test-market new products and to assist in corporate cash flow. Because of his audiologic background, Barry was chosen to operate the dispensary. But the American Speech and Hearing Association (ASHA) had long decreed that dispensing hearing aids, by a member, was unethical, and it roundly drummed Barry out of the organization (which in those days was tantamount to ejecting you from the profession). But Barry persisted, and soon other individuals holding a long pent-up concern that ASHA's ethical code was not helpful to the profession began to exert pressure on ASHA to change its ethical stance. It took some time, but in 1979 the ASHA Code of Ethics was finally modified to permit the dispensing of aids.

Nowadays the dispensing of hearing aids and other amplification devices is such a cornerstone of the profession that we have to be reminded of what it was like before the ASHA code was changed. After you had spent hours in audiometric testing and the evaluation of several aids, you could only send the client off to a hearing aid dealer whose code of ethics was less burdensome. It was very unlikely that you would ever see that client again. You never really knew whether they had even acquired an aid or whether they were successful users. There was very little feedback and no accountability. Only in the VA and the military clinics, where the audiologist was permitted to be the dispenser, did the audiologist have any sense of closure, any feel for the ultimate consequences of his or her work. It is fair to say that, today, audiology is a very different profession as a result of Barry's defection leading to that pivotal decision by ASHA in 1979. It provided a key part of the framework for the rise of private practice, a development so essential to the viability of an independent profession.

Assistive Devices

Audiologists have long been familiar with FM systems employing remote microphones, and tend to equate these with all assistive listening devices (ALDs). But Cynthia Compton Conley (Figure 6–12), of Gallaudet University, reminds us that there are a wide variety of devices designed to improve the communication skills, the well-being, and the quality of life of hearing- impaired and deafened persons, and that not all such devices involve "listening." Thus, although the term ALD is still being used, a more appropriate umbrella

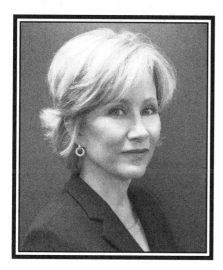

Figure 6–12. Cynthia Compton Conley. (Courtesy of Gallaudet University.)

term, hearing assistance technology (HAT), refers to both auditory and nonauditory assistive technology. Historically, the first were alerting devices, designed to assist the individual to be aware of and identify environmental sounds and relevant or dangerous situations. These include systems that flash a light or vibrate a transducer when the doorbell rings, when the baby cries, and so forth.

A second category of assistive devices includes systems to assist in telephone communication, for example, devices to amplify the telephone signal.

Third are devices to assist in the enjoyment of broadcast and other media. In these systems, the audio signal from the broadcast source is amplified and delivered to the hearing-impaired person either via a hardwired amplification system, such as coupling a portable music player to one's hearing aids or implant via direct audio input or induction, or via wireless transmission. The wireless, devices may be of three types: (1) Infrared (IR), (2) FM carrier, or (3) induction (audio loop). Each of these systems consists of a transmitter and a wireless receiver. Although the transmitter can be connected to the sound source via a microphone, usually the transmitter is simply plugged into the sound source directly.

The history of remote-microphone technology can be traced back to the availability of the very first commercially available vacuum tubes in the 1920s. In 1949 Leland Watson and Thomas Tolan, in their comprehensive volume, *Hearing Tests and Hearing Instruments*, noted that, in the early 1930s multiple vacuum tube hearing aids were widely installed in schools for the deaf, leagues for the hard of hearing, churches, and theaters. Foreshadowing the later development of the wireless remote microphone, a microphone was placed in close proximity to the source of sound (loudspeaker or live speaker) and hard wired to the multiple aids. To their amazement hearing-impaired listeners found that, in churches and theaters, they could hear as well, and sometimes even better, than their normally hearing neighbors. They reported that it was as if they were seated directly in front of the sound source. For them, the sound source was not weakened by distance, reflections, or echoes as it would be for normally hearing persons.

The first truly practical individual remote microphone devices were introduced in 1969–1970 by both the Williams Sound company and the Phonic Ear Company. The Williams Sound system used a modified AM radio and operated in the commercial AM band. After the FCC approved the 72- to 76-MHz FM band, in the early 1970s, Phonic Ear introduced the well-known COMTEK system which transmitted at 72 MHz.

Both research and clinical experience have shown that there are many listening situations in which ALDs give better results than conventional hearing aids. They do so by the simple expedient of moving the microphone from the ear of the listener to the mouth of the talker, thereby improving the signal-to-competing-background-noise ratio at the listener's ear. ALDs have proven particularly helpful for elderly persons who do not benefit optimally from conventional aids, and for children suspected of auditory processing disorder. As ALD technology advances to include improvements in FM technology and the advancement of newer technologies such as Bluetooth, we may anticipate greater acceptance of these devices by both audiologists and their clients.

Cochlear Implants

In the United States, cochlear implants were pioneered in the early 1960s by, William House at the House Ear Institute in Los Ange-les, F. Blair Simmons, at Stanford University, Michael Merzenich and Robin Michelson at the University of California/San Francisco (UCSF), and Donald Eddington at the University of Utah. Early models were essentially single-channel devices, employing a unitary implanted electrode that provided virtually no "place" or spectral information. But to many peoples' surprise just the information in the temporal envelope of the speech waveform seemed to provide useful cues for speech understanding in severely and profoundly hearing-impaired individuals. At this early stage, however, there were many doubters and skeptics. Some even suggested that implanting electrodes in the cochlea of a living patient was tantamount to human experimentation.

In an effort to resolve these concerns, and to provide objective evidence for or against cochlear implantation, the National Institute of Communicative Disorders and Stroke (NINCDS) in 1975 awarded a contract to a highly regarded hearing scientist, the late Robert Bilger, then at the University of Pittsburgh, to systematically evaluate a group of 13 profoundly hearing-impaired individuals who had received single-channel implants. At the outset of the study, Bilger was skeptical about cochlear implants, but, at its conclusion, emerged as a reluctant supporter as his data showed clear evidence that, in this study group, cochlear implants appeared to provide more useful information than conventional hearing aids. Bilger's 1976 report is widely viewed as a significant turning point in the history of cochlear implantation, largely because of the great respect that Bilger enjoyed among audiologists, otolaryngologists, and hearing scientists. The way was now cleared for the subsequent development of multichannel devices.

One of the most successful multiple electrode systems has been the Nucleus device, originally developed by Graeme Clark

(Figure 6–13) and his team at the University of Melbourne, Australia in the 1970s, and first implanted in the United States at the University of Iowa. Another successful device is the Clarion unit, developed as a result of scientific effort led by the group at UCSF.

The progress of cochlear implants over the past three decades has been truly remarkable. The early systems were essentially aids to lip reading. Few users could maintain a conversation without the aid of visual cues. But as the number of electrodes increased, and speech coding strategies became more sophisticated, performance in the "auditory only" condition has improved several fold. It is now quite reasonable to expect that a suitably chosen candidate will be able to converse easily over the telephone. Thirty years ago, few would have predicted that this level of performance would ever be attainable. Much of this success is the result of painstaking research and clinical effort by, among others, Carolyn Brown, Michael Dorman, Bruce Ganz, Ann Geers, Josef Miller, Richard Miyamota, Mary Jo Osberger, Charles

Parkins, Robert Shannon, Margo Skinner, Mario Svirsky, and Richard Tyler.

Although the bulk of research on patients with cochlear implants has been confined to behavioral studies involving various dimensions of speech perception, auditory evoked potentials have proven quite useful in the evaluation of both children and adults. Individuals who have exploited auditory evoked responses to great advantage in this area are Nina Kraus, of Northwestern University, Paul Kileny (Figure 6–14), of the University of Michigan, and Paul Abbas and Carolyn Brown, of the University of Iowa.

Although the importance of successful surgical placement of the electrodes within the cochlea cannot be overestimated, the major share of the credit for the present status of cochlear implants surely must go to those researchers who have patiently and methodically improved the speech coding strategies, and to the audiologists who have provided the lengthy, often tedious, aural rehabilitation sessions so critical to the successful use of cochlear implants.

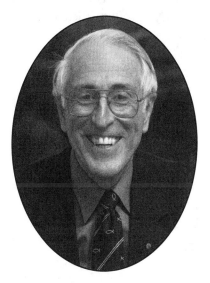

Figure 6–13. Graeme Clark. (Courtesy of the Bionic Ear Institute.)

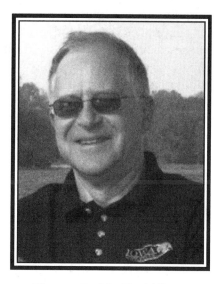

Figure 6–14. Paul Kileny.

Auditory Training

The steady rise of cochlear implants has been responsible for much of the resurgence of interest in auditory training. Very early in the history of cochlear implants, it became increasingly clear that their efficacy was very much enhanced by a program of systematic auditory training following implantation. Audiologists had long paid lip service to the idea that the value of a wearable hearing aid could be enhanced by auditory training, but only a few (the late Elmer Owens at UCSF comes to mind) pursued the possibilities vigorously. But from the very first patient implanted with a single-channel device, the dramatic value of a rigorous program of post-surgical aural rehabilitation was evident. The success of the auditory training programs developed to meet this need have, quite appropriately, sparked a resurgence of interest in all applications of systematic auditory training.

Attempts to exploit the residual hearing of severely and profoundly hearing-impaired persons have a history much longer than audiology. Long before there were audiometers and hearing aids, educators of the deaf were at the front lines of auditory training, using whatever tools were available. Alexander Graham Bell, inventor of the telephone and founder of the AG Bell Association, took a special interest in the possibilities of auditory training because of his wife's hearing loss. He was a strong proponent of the aural approach and lent his considerable reputation to its promulgation in the last quarter of the 19th century. Another early supporter of systematic training in listening was Max Goldstein who founded the world-famous Central Institute for the Deaf in St. Louis.

But it was the advent of World War II, and the military aural rehabilitation programs that mark the beginning of the modern era in auditory training. At Deshon General Hospital, for example, Raymond Carhart developed an 8-week individualized therapy program emphasizing critical listening, precise and rapid recognition of phonetic elements, re-establishment of the recognition of familiar noises, and training in auditory discrimination under adverse listening conditions. Similar programs were initiated at the other centers as the war wound down. The efforts were popular with the veterans who experienced the programs, but after the war enthusiasm for auditory training as a supplement to hearing aid use slowly waned. There were a number of reasons for this decline: the two most important were lack of third-party reimbursement for such training and lack of empirical evidence of its efficacy. However, dedicated professionals like Mark Ross (Figure 6–15), who as a World War II veteran passed through a wartime program, and Norman Erber continued to research and develop training programs.

Beginning in the 1980s, however, renewed broad interest in auditory training was stimulated by two research thrusts: (1) maximizing the value of cochlear implants, and (2) carefully controlled efficacy studies. The impact of cochlear implants on the resurgence of auditory training was amplified in

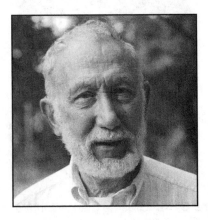

Figure 6–15. Mark Ross.

the previous section. Relative to efficacy, a ground breaking study at Walter Reed Army Hospital by Brian Walden and colleagues in 1981 demonstrated the value of a comprehensive analytic auditory training program emphasizing consonant discrimination in young hearing-impaired adults. In 1996 Patricia Kricos (Figure 6–16) and Alice Holmes reported results of a very well-controlled study in which they compared the efficacy of a bottom-up analytic approach with a more top-down synthetic approach to auditory training. In 2005, however, Robert Sweetow (Figure 6–17) and Catherine Palmer (Figure 6–18) carried out a comprehensive review of the auditory training literature and found very little convincing evidence of genuine efficacy.

Interestingly, both Walden et al. and Kricos and Holmes questioned the value of an analytic approach in the case of elderly hearing aid users. Because elderly persons are the majority of hearing aid users, this conclusion, based on careful research, has been of more than passing interest to the developers of auditory training programs. Some have suggested that, over the years, Carhart's emphasis on "critical listening" and "precise and rapid recognition of phonetic elements"

has led to an overemphasis on an analytic as opposed to a more synthetic approach to auditory training. Perhaps, they reason, an auditory training regimen focused on consonant discrimination drills is likely to be less effective with elderly persons than a more synthetic approach, emphasizing coping strategies, development of good listening habits, concentration on the meaning of messages, and nonverbal and situational cues.

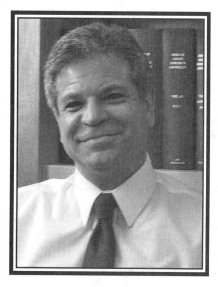

Figure 6–17. Robert Sweetow.

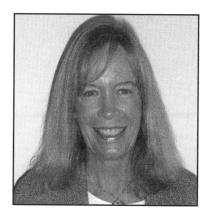

Figure 6–16. Pat Kricos. (Courtesy of University of Florida.)

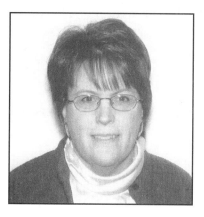

Figure 6–18. Catherine Palmer.

Much of the current enthusiasm for auditory training derives from relatively recent studies by neuroscientists of neural plasticity, especially in the auditory system. There is convincing evidence that concentrated auditory stimulation can alter neural organization throughout the auditory system. Moreover, Nina Kraus and Kelly Tremblay have shown that neurophysiologic changes produced by auditory training actually generalize to other stimuli not specifically targeted for training. They have even shown changes in the P1, N1, and P2 components of the auditory evoked response after systematic auditory training.

Perhaps the most significant development for the future of auditory training has been the recent emergence of self-paced, self-instructional materials, sometimes in the form of interactive games. Thanks to computer technology, programs designed to improve auditory discrimination and phonemic awareness, and to enhance language learning, can be pursued at school, at the office, at home, or in any other environment where computer facilities are available.

In summary, auditory training flowered immediately after World War II, then almost faded from sight for the next three decades. Within the past two decades, however, we have seen a strong resurgence of research and the clinical application of auditory training, influenced greatly by its successful use in cochlear implant rehabilitation and by the demonstration of neural plasticity in the auditory system. In their excellent historical review, Kricos and Holmes make the profound point that auditory training may be: the most powerful, yet underutilized, tool at the audiologist's disposal.

Clear Speech

Before there were hearing aids and assistive devices, there was clear speech. This very old idea, that hearing-impaired individuals find it helpful if the speaker pronounces slowly and distinctly, has enjoyed a resurgence of interest in recent years. Especially noteworthy have been the research studies on the effects of slowing speech rate, improving enunciation, emphasizing key words, and inserting pauses at clause boundaries. Among the many individuals who have contributed to recent research on clear speech, the contributions of Louis Braida at MIT, Dianne Kewley-Port at Indiana University, Sarah Ferguson at the University of Kansas, Karen Helfer at the University of Massachusetts, and Nancy Tye-Murray at CID-Washington University have been particularly interesting.

7

Pediatric Audiology

Audiologists have long been aware of the special considerations required when dealing with babies and young children suspected of hearing loss. Because the period from infancy to about 14 years is marked by substantial developmental changes, techniques for detecting and assessing hearing loss in the pediatric population are, necessarily, critically dependent on the child's chronological age. It is useful, in this regard to discuss separately (1) the screening of newborn and very young infants in order to detect hearing loss, and (2) the special problems of assessing the nature and degree of hearing loss in children in the age range from 3 years to 8 or 9 years.

Screening in Newborn Babies and Infants

Individuals who worked with hearing-impaired and deaf children were long aware of the critical importance of early detection of loss for subsequent language development and academic achievement. Thus, efforts to screen young children for hearing loss have a long history. But the behavioral tools available for screening in the early years of the profession were not totally satisfactory. They included observation of head turning in response to common environmental sounds and conditioning paradigms that ranged from simple to complex. Techniques employing unconditioned responses to sound, often termed Play Audiometry or Behavioral Observation Audiometry (BOA), were popular from the 1930s until well into the 1970s. While one tester engaged the child in some form of play activity, another tester presented sounds from various directions and observed whether the child made an appropriate turning response. Five persistent problems plagued these approaches. First, over the age range from 0 to 12 months the normal infant's ability to localize sounds accurately and swiftly undergoes significant maturation; second, one could not always be sure of the reliability of the child's behavioral responses; third, habituation to the sounds could be very rapid; fourth, deciding whether an appropriate response had occurred involved a good deal of subjective judgment on the part of the examiners; and, fifth, screening children in the important age range from 0 to 3 years was always a bit dicey. Crying, squirming, thrashing about, and falling asleep were serious impediments to successful behavioral testing.

To counter these persistent problems, some clinicians turned to what were, in that period, often described as "objective" techniques. Chief among these were, in the 1940s and 1950s, the electrodermal response (EDR), in the 1950s the Heart Rate Response (HRR), in the 1960s Respiration Audiometry, in the 1970s the Crib-O-Gram, and in the 1980s the Auditory Response Cradle. All were plagued by significant problems and were never adopted on a widespread basis.

But the advent of the auditory brainstem response, or ABR, and otoacoustic emissions, opened up the playing field substantially. These two techniques made it possible, for the first time, to screen babies literally from the moment of birth with techniques whose reliability could be tested and affirmed. It seemed that the screening of all babies born in the United States (i.e., genuine universal screening) might, indeed, be feasible.

The single individual who has had the greatest impact on the concept of universal screening of newborn babies is certainly Marion Downs (Figure 7–1) of the University of Colorado. She founded the first screening program in Colorado in 1962, and has never ceased to push for universal screening of every newborn. Few have been so devoted to an audiologic cause.

Because the ABR is virtually completely independent of the state of wakefulness or sleep of babies, it seemed a likely candidate

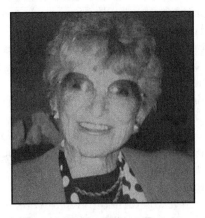

Figure 7–1. Marion Downs.

for screening babies of all ages, but it was not until the publication of a seminal paper by Kurt Hecox and Robert Galambos in 1971 that the value of ABR in the evaluation of the pediatric population began to be accepted by the pediatric audiologic community. Today it is difficult to imagine the evaluation of newborns, infants, and young children without ABR, but before this important paper appeared, behavioral techniques, many of extremely questionable validity, were the rule. The paper by Hecox and Galambos stirred the pot, and the extraordinary value of ABR in the evaluation of infants and young children soon became evident.

Nevertheless, it was difficult to reconcile the magnitude of universal individual screening with what was perceived to be the excessive cost of individual ABR testing. The false positive rate was low but the procedure was perceived to be too expensive for widespread use.

A more likely candidate appeared on the scene with the advent of transient evoked otoacoustic emissions (TEOAE). A series of pioneering studies at the Women and Infants Hospital of Rhode Island by a team led by Karl White (Figure 7–2), of Utah State University and Thomas Behrens of the United States Department of Education showed that TEOAEs could be used to screen babies quite successfully and at moderate cost. The only problem here was the perception that the false positive rate of TEOAE screening (variously estimated at 10–20%) was prohibitive. Well, if ABR had a low false positive rate but was too expensive, and TEOAE had a high false positive rate but was less expensive, then the idea quickly took hold that the ideal solution was a two-stage process in which TEOAEs are obtained on every baby in the first stage, and ABR is used in the second stage, but only on those babies who failed the first stage. All of this led to an NIH

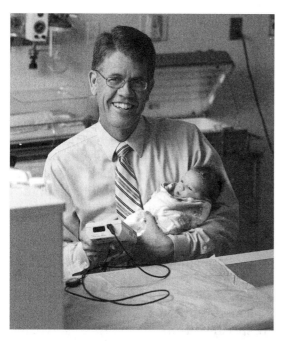

Figure 7–2. Karl White. (Courtesy of Utah State University Public Relations and Marketing.)

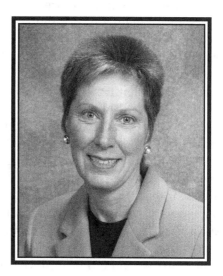

Figure 7–3. Deborah Hayes. (Courtesy of the Children's Hospital of Denver.)

Consensus Conference on Newborn Screening in 1993 in which just such a two-stage program for screening was recommended. At this writing, screening programs based on this and similar models have now been successfully organized in every state and the District of Columbia. Most are mandated by state legislation: the remainder are supported by local Public Health Departments. We can count this as one of the major achievements of our profession.

In the pediatric research arena, both Judy Widen, at the University of Kansas, and Susan Norton, at the University of Washington, have made important contributions to the evaluation of screening protocols and screening technology. In addition, Deborah Hayes (Figure 7–3), of the Denver Children's Hospital, has been a tireless worker in educating pediatricians, otolaryngologists, and other medical specialists on the impor-

tance of early detection and the provision of comprehensive services to hearing-impaired infants, children, and their parents.

Assessing Young Children

Successful intervention in hearing-impaired children is greatly facilitated by detailed knowledge of the audiometric contours and levels of speech understanding on the two ears. In the age range from about 5 to 36 months, play audiometric techniques began to give way, in the 1950s and 1960s to conditioning paradigms in which appropriate behavioral responses to sounds were systematically reinforced. Examples were Visual Reinforcement Audiometry (VRA), the Conditioned Orienting Response (COR), Tangible Reinforcement Operant Conditioning

Audiometry (TROCA), and Conditioned Play Audiometry (CPA). All continue in use today, in spite of the inherent limitations of behavioral responses in young children, because they provide, in many cases, rapid and efficient frequency-specific and ear-specific information about sensitivity loss.

Assessing speech understanding in the pediatric population has, itself, a long and interesting history. As the value of the spondee and PB words lists in the evaluation of hearing-impaired adults became evident in the late 1940s, a similar approach in pediatric evaluation seemed inevitable. But it was equally clear that children lacked the vocabulary necessary to deal with many of the words in these lists. Harriet Haskins, then a student in Carhart's program at Northwestern University, was the first to develop, in 1949, words lists within the vocabulary of children as young as 5 years. They were called the PB-K lists, to indicate that they were suitable for the average kindergartner, and they are still in use today.

But the problems of translating speech audiometry to the pediatric population extended beyond the suitability of the materials. Especially in the youngest age range, from 3 to 6 years, the ever present problems of immature cognitive skills, habituation, reliability of response, and so forth required the development of techniques of administration appropriate for young children. Generally, these have taken the form of a closed-set, picture-pointing paradigm based on two important considerations, receptive language ability and response set definition. The child hears a word or sentence, and then points to one of a small number of pictures illustrating the word or sentence. One of the first successful tests of this genre was the Word Intelligibility by Picture Identification (WIPI) test, developed by Ross and Lerman in 1970. In 1980 Elliott and Katz offered the Northwestern University Children's Perception of Speech (NU-CHIPS) test, employing monosyllabic words known to be in the vocabulary of children more than 2½ years old. Both employed a closed-set response mode, but task domain was unrestricted in the sense that targets and foils could be interchanged across many different response sets. In the late 1970s, Susan Jerger took a different approach in the development of the Pediatric Speech Intelligibility (PSI) test. The test employs picture-pointing responses to both words and sentences in the presence of a competing speech message. Here the words and sentences were actually generated by normal children in the age range from 3 to 6 years of age. The PSI test employs a closed-set response mode, but the task domain is restricted in the sense that targets are specified. Throughout the decades of the 1980s and 1990s, important enhancements to pediatric speech testing techniques have been contributed by, among many others, Arthur Boothroyd, Harry Levitt, Laurie Eisenberg, David Pisoni, Richard Seewald, and Karen Kirk.

A particularly dramatic example of how basic research can impact clinical practice is the extent to which Harry Levitt's classic 1970 paper on adaptive testing protocols "Transformed Up and Down Methods in Psychoacoustics" has permeated speech intelligibility testing in both adults and children. The Quick Speech-in-Noise (QuickSIN) test and the Hearing-in-Noise Test (HINT); both based on the adaptive techniques outlined in Levitt's paper, have taken advantage of the greater efficiency offered by this approach in their speech intelligibility test procedures.

Within the past decade, we have seen renewed interest in combining auditory and visual stimuli in pediatric evaluation. As early as 1972 Ross and Lerman, using the WIPI test, compared scores obtained via auditory-alone presentation with scores obtained via combined auditory and visual presentation.

But in that period, synchronization of the auditory and visual representations was technically difficult unless the presentation was live. In recent years, however, with the development of computerized presentation of digitized auditory and visual stimuli, interest in this approach has expanded. Arthur Boothroyd, A. Martinez, Karen Kirk, David Pisoni, Laurie Eisenberg, Susan Jerger, and Nancy Tye-Murray are currently active in this arena. Of particular current interest is the work of Boothroyd, Eisenberg, and Martinez on speech pattern contrast perception in both auditory-only and auditory-visual modes using computerized tasks (OLIMSPAC and VIPSPAC).

One of the positive dividends of the earlier identification of mild to severe hearing loss as a result of infant screening programs has been the opportunity to gather previously scarce data on the development of language and literacy in these children. As early as the 1970s, Julia Davis and her associates at the University of Iowa, called attention to the gaps in our knowledge of reading, language, and academic achievement in this population. Recent advances in this area have been well summarized in a report by Mary Pat Moeller, J. Bruce Tomblin, Christine Yoshinaga-Itano, Carol Connor, and Susan Jerger.

8

Auditory Processing Disorder

In the late 1940s, Helmer Myklebust (Figure 8–1), a psychologist with a background of interest in deaf children, opened a diagnostic children's hearing clinic at Northwestern University's School of Speech and encouraged parents, pediatricians, and other professionals to refer children suspected of possible hearing loss. The primary presenting symptom that brought children to the clinic, and indeed to most hearing-care professionals in that era, was "not talking" (i.e., failure to develop speech appropriate to the child's chronologic age), an inevitable consequence of moderate to severe hearing loss. Myklebust found such losses in the majority of the children referred to the clinic. But he also noted that many of the children referred for lack of appropriate speech development had no obvious hearing loss. Myklebust thought that some of these children might have a form of mild auditory agnosia. He noted that they seemed to have a specifically "listening" problem. They didn't seem to be able to direct their attention to relevant sounds. Their auditory environment consisted of many individuals sounds, all of equal importance. They did not seem to be able to bring relevant sounds to the foreground and irrelevant sounds to the background. Their auditory world, said Myklebust, was "conglomerate."

To fit these children into a coherent framework Myklebust introduced the term "auditory disorder" as a descriptor covering not only peripheral hearing loss but problems at higher levels in the auditory system, especially as they affected language development. He then developed a systematic behavioral approach to the differential diagnosis of such disorders.

A number of audiologists in the United States thought that the development of "sensitized speech testing" by the Italians under Ettore Bocca in the 1950s had important implications for the diagnosis of such "central auditory disorders." The work of the Italians had been based on patients with temporal lobe tumors, but the intuitive leap to the assessment of persons with auditory complaints, but lacking "hard" neurologic signs,

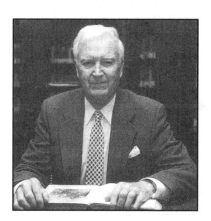

Figure 8–1. Helmer Myklebust.

was irresistible. Several investigators set out to devise difficult or "sensitized" speech audiometric tasks. Chief among these were tests involving dichotic listening.

The work on ear and hemisphere asymmetries by Brenda Milner and Doreen Kimura, at McGill University in Montreal, generated an interest in the development of dichotic listening tests that might prove useful in evaluating adults with brain lesions, and by extension, children with "auditory disorders."

Over the next two decades, a number of dichotic tests or test batteries were developed for clinical use. In 1962 Jack Katz developed the staggered spondee word (SSW) test. A pair of spondee words is presented dichotically, but the second syllable of one word overlaps the first syllable of the other. Scoring and interpretation are complex. Jack Willeford, in 1977, developed a dichotic sentence test using natural sentences. The procedure was used effectively by Lynn and Gilroy in their 1977 comprehensive study of adults with verified brain lesions. During that same period, Berlin et al. developed a dichotic test procedure based on consonant-vowel (CV) nonsense syllables. Copies of the Berlin tapes were widely used worldwide for the next 30 years. During the decade of the 1970s, Susan Jerger and James Jerger modified the synthetic sentence identification (SSI) paradigm by adding either an ipsilateral (SSI-ICM) or a contralateral (SSI-CCM) competing message. In 1983 a dichotic version of the SSI sentences, the dichotic sentence identification (DSI) test was developed by Fifer (Figure 8–2), Jerger, Berlin, Tobey, and Campbell.

It should be emphasized that much of this early development of dichotic testing was focused on the study of adults, usually with *verified brain lesions*. Beginning in the late 1970s, however, interest turned toward

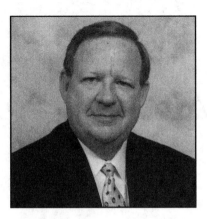

Figure 8–2. Robert Fifer.

children. Could "sensitized" speech testing, and especially dichotic testing, be used to evaluate children suspected of auditory processing disorder (APD)?

Although dichotic tests have played a major role in APD assessment, other approaches have included low-pass filtering, compressed or speeded speech, temporal and frequency patterning, and gap detection.

During the 1980s, the idea that some children might have particular problems with the processing of auditory input in spite of normal sensitivity spread rapidly. Although Myklebust had raised the issue three decades earlier, the burgeoning societal interest in reading problems, language delay, learning disability, and attention deficit disorder stimulated a widespread rebirth of the concept. Initial impetus came from a landmark publication, "The Psychopathology and Education of the Brain-Injured Child," by psycho-educational consultants Alfred Strauss and Laura Lehtinen in 1947. The authors proposed a straightforward definition. A child with organic impairment of the brain, sustained either before, during, or after birth, may show disturbances in perception, thinking, and emotional behavior. Such disturbances prevent or impede the normal process of learning. They can be demonstrated by "specific tests."

In this concise definition, prepared more than 60 years ago, one can discern much of the current rationale for the diagnosis and treatment of children suspected of a broad variety of disorders including APD. The overriding theme of this approach was "learning disability." The child was targeted for evaluation because of an assumed learning problem, usually reflected in poor academic performance. The first methodological approach to Strauss and Lehtinens' claim that such disturbances could be demonstrated by specific tests was the development of the Illinois Test of Psycholinguistic Abilities (ITPA) by Sam Kirk in1968. Kirk defined a number of theoretical constructs thought to underlie the communication skills necessary for adequate learning. In the perceptual-motor domain the ITPA contained five auditory subtests:

Auditory Reception

Auditory Association

Auditory Sequential Memory

Auditory Closure

Sound Blending

Poor performance on one or more these subtests was assumed to be consistent with an auditory perceptual problem. Here we can see the earliest stages of development of one popular contemporary view of auditory processing disorder shared by many audiologists and speech-language pathologists. Auditory perception is viewed as the summation of a number of discrete, measurable abilities. More recently, several additional hypothesized discrete abilities have been added to Kirk's original list.

Divergence Begins

One can discern the development of three quite different approaches to the concept of auditory processing disorder: the first might be called the "audiologic" approach; the second the "psycho-educational" approach, and the third, the "language processing" approach.

The Audiologic Approach

The audiologic approach built on the earlier observations that persons with brain injury affecting the auditory central nervous system exhibited certain behaviors; ergo, if tests revealed these same behaviors, then a link to brain injury was established. Several investigators set out to devise tests of the desired behavior appropriate for children.

Based both on the dichotic listening model and on the earlier work of Ettore Boca, Robert Keith (Figure 8–3), of the University of Cincinnati developed, early in the 1980s,

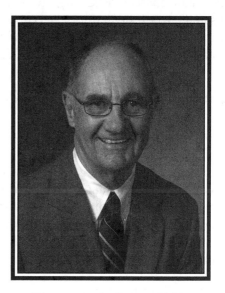

Figure 8–3. Robert Keith.

a screening test battery appropriate for children suspected of APD. His SCAN–C test is presently the most widely used test battery in this arena. It includes both dichotic competing word and dichotic competing sentence subtests along with two degraded speech subtests of filtered words and speech in noise. Later Keith developed an adult version, SCAN-A, based on the same general principles upon which SCAN-C had been developed.

Willeford's battery, including his competing sentences test and Katz' SSW procedure have also been widely applied to children with apparently poor listening skills. In 1983 Susan Jerger, James Jerger, and Sam Abrams showed that, on the ipsilateral and contralateral competing message conditions of the Pediatric Speech Intelligibility Test (PSI), the performance of children suspected of APD closely resembled the performance of children with verified brain lesions.

The rationale for most of these procedures might be summarized as follows. If persons with known injury to the auditory nervous system perform in a characteristic way on these tests, then if a child performs in that same characteristic way, an injury to that same part of the auditory nervous system may be assumed. The validity of this rationale has rarely been tested in children.

The Psycho-Educational Approach

The psycho-educational approach, on the other hand, is built on the premise of a set of primary auditory abilities that are measurable by appropriate techniques. This approach is illustrated by the auditory skills subtests of the 1974 Goldman, Fristoe, Woodcock Scale. This instrument posited four dimensions of auditory perceptual processing:

Auditory Discrimination

Auditory Memory

Auditory Selective Attention

Sound-Symbol Association

Other investigators have suggested additional dimensions, but they are all variations on the theme of hypothesized discrete perceptual processes. Teri Bellis (Figure 8–4), in 1996, uniquely, combined an audiologic approach to testing within a framework of five discrete dimensions of processing.

The idea that auditory processing ability underlies other basic abilities such as language development and reading was a natural outgrowth of the schema laid out so clearly by Strauss and Lehtinen. If learning is based on language, and if language is learned primarily through the auditory modality, then it is reasonable to suppose that problems in auditory perceptual processing could lead to problems in language acquisition and to subsequent learning disability. Christine Sloan was an early advocate of this position.

Paula Tallal and her colleagues were among the first to investigate the area system-

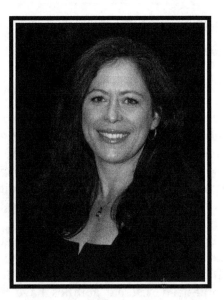

Figure 8–4. Teri Bellis. (Courtesy of RC Photographic productions.)

atically. Their early studies of children with language delay suggested that some showed: a specific problem in responding to either verbal or nonverbal rapidly changing stimuli. Here is a suggestion that the number of primary auditory perceptual abilities underlying the auditory processing abilities which, in turn, underlie successful language development, may be limited in number. Tallal and colleagues have developed sophisticated techniques for evaluating and treating disorders of "rapid auditory processing," or RAP.

Recently, a group of Australian investigators, led by Sharon Cameron (Figure 8–5), have suggested that a different unitary aspect of auditory perception, the ability to differentiate spatially dissimilar foreground and background sounds, might be present in a high proportion of children at risk for APD. This is eerily reminiscent of Myklebust's original description of a fundamental problem in resolving auditory foreground and background.

The Language Processing Approach

Gradually, the initial emphasis on auditory processing has, in some circles, become an emphasis on language processing. People whose primary interest is childhood language disorders, particularly their management, emphasize that auditory processing is only one component of the processing of language in difficult acoustic environments. In other words, factors other than auditory perceptual disorder may contribute to what many have identified as symptoms of APD, and that they may interact with auditory perceptual disorders to complicate language processing.

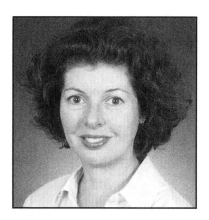

Figure 8–5. Sharon Cameron.

It is certainly the case that auditory processing disorder (APD) has come to mean different things to different people! It began as a fairly circumscribed perceptual concept —difficulty in separating auditory foreground from auditory background in children—but it has morphed along divergent paths. One path was developed by audiologists, initially studying brain-injured adults, then applying these findings to the testing of children. A second path was developed by psycho-educational specialists based on the concept of discrete auditory perceptual abilities, a paradigm subsequently adopted by many audiologists and speech-language pathologists as a model for diagnosing and treating disorders of auditory processing. A third path has been traced by persons primarily interested in the complex interactions among auditory processing disorder and other cognitive dimensions as they impact language acquisition and learning.

Only the future student of APD history will be able to record whether these paths continue to diverge, or whether they eventually begin to converge on a more unitary conceptualization of, and approach to, the APD problem.

9

Tinnitus Evaluation and Therapy

Tinnitus researcher Gary Jacobson (Figure 9–1) reports that the prevalence of tinnitus in the United States is estimated to be as much as 40 million individuals. Of this number, an estimated 7 to 8 million find it sufficiently bothersome that they seek medical care. Of this number, an estimated 2 million find it so distressing that they are virtually disabled. Yet for many years surprisingly few audiologists engaged the problem from the standpoint of either clinical or research interest. The history of tinnitus research has been studied extensively by James Henry of the National Center for Research in Audi-tory Rehabilitation (NCRAR) at the Portland VA Medical Center He has traced it back to the early 19th century. Jean Marc Gaspard Itard (famous as the author of *The Wild Boy of Aveyron*) was the Chief Physician at the National Institute for Deaf-Mutes in Paris, and is often credited as the founder of oto-rhino-laryngology and of the concept of special education. In 1821 he observed that, in his deaf pupils (some of whom surely had less than total losses), tinnitus could be treated with masking sounds and that the pitch of the tinnitus was related to the optimal masking sound.

Over the years, many individuals attempted to refine this observation by developing psychoacoustic measures of the loudness and pitch of tinnitus. Among the early attempts were the studies of R. L Wegel (of audiometer fame) and E. M. Josephson in 1931. Both attempted to measure the loudness and pitch of the tinnitus by means of pure tones. Wegel, moreover, generated tinnitus masking curves by noting the levels at which tonal maskers of different frequencies just masked the tinnitus. Later in the decade, Edmund Prince Fowler (of audiogram fame) adapted his binaural loudness balance test to the measurement of tinnitus by having the patient match the pitch and intensity of

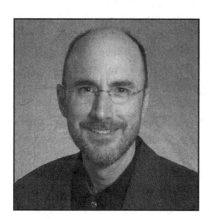

Figure 9–1. Gary Jacobson. (Courtesy of Anne Rayner.)

the tinnitus in one ear with the pitch and intensity of an actual tone in the opposite ear. Using this technique, Fowler reported that, although the patient might describe the tinnitus as "very loud," it was actually matched by a tone at a sensation level of only 5 to 10 dB. Fowler's conclusion, that tinnitus was an "illusion" that tended to be exaggerated, was to be reasserted by many subsequent investigators.

The patient's ability to describe his or her tinnitus has often been a problem. Investigators first attempted to find a pure tone frequency on the audiometer that matched the tinnitus, but immediately encountered problems. A major source of the difficulty was the fact that tinnitus takes many forms; in some a ringing sound much like a very high-frequency pure tone, but in others more like a narrow or broad band noise. Early pioneers in tinnitus evaluation included Victor Goodhill at UCLA, Jack Vernon, Robert Johnson, and Mary Meikle at the Oregon Health Sciences University Hearing Research Center, Richard Tyler at the University of Iowa, and M. J. Penner at the University of Maryland. Much of this work concerned attempts to characterize tinnitus by psychoacoustic measures, but for a variety of reasons. there are still no standardized tests to characterize tinnitus. James Henry (Figure 9–2), points out that, although part of the problem is lack of confidence in the reliability of some psychoacoustic measures, a principal source of delay is the conflict between the psychoacoustician's desire for rigorous measurement technique and the clinician's desire for a realistic procedure that patients can perform in a reasonable amount of time.

Another approach to the problem has been the development of tinnitus questionnaires. Several have been developed based on differing approaches: among the most popular are the Tinnitus Handicap Questionnaire, developed by Kuk, Tyler, and Russell;

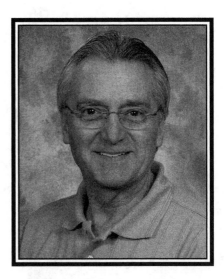

Figure 9–2. James Henry.

the Tinnitus Handicap Inventory, developed by Newman and Jacobson; and the Tinnitus Cognitions Questionnaire developed by Wilson and Henry. But, again, there is little standardization in this arena. Recognizing the need for more standardization in the interest of comparing results across clinics and across treatment options, a number of tinnitus investigators agreed to meet in an attempt to reach a consensus on matters relating to the evaluation and treatment of tinnitus. The first Tinnitus Research Initiative meeting was held in Regensburg, Germany in 2006. The United States was represented by A. Cacace, M. Meikle, J. Melcher, and J. P. Rauschecker. Considering the long history of contention on so many matters relating to tinnitus, the group managed to make substantial progress in defining needs and establishing some protocols. In other areas, especially psychophysical measures of tinnitus, agreement continued to be elusive.

The discovery that tinnitus could be purposely masked to provide relief to the sufferer is credited to Harald Feldmann of Germany. In 1971 he found that tinnitus could be inhibited by an externally presented sound in 89% of tinnitus sufferers. He noted, moreover, that inhibition of the tinnitus sometimes remained for a period of time after cessation of the masker (later termed "residual inhibition" by Jack Vernon). These findings have been successfully exploited by means of tinnitus masking devices, worn much like a behind-the-ear hearing aid. Many of the benefits derived from tinnitus masking are also realized through the use of conventional hearing aids.

Within the past two decades, the number of other treatment options for tinnitus has expanded considerably. Drug treatments include antidepressants, acamprosate, zinc, gabapentin, lidocaine, antioxidants, minerals, vitamins and herbs, and melatonin. Cognitive therapy treatments include the Tinnitus Retraining therapy of Jasterboff, and the Tinnitus Activities treatment of Tyler, Gogel, and Gehringer. Clinical trials of these various treatment options have been scarce. A notable exception was a very carefully controlled 2006 study by James Henry, Martin Schechter, Tara Zaugg, Susan Griest, Pawel Jasterboff, Jack Vernon, Christine Kaelin, Mary Meikle, Karen Lyons, and Barbara Stewart. They compared the outcomes of two treatments, tinnitus masking and tinnitus retraining therapy. Results showed that, when the degree of tinnitus was severe, the decline in tinnitus following treatment was greater after tinnitus retraining therapy than after tinnitus masking. But when the degree of tinnitus was only moderate, both treatments produced about the same decline in tinnitus.

Much has been learned about the troubling malady of tinnitus over the past two decades, but it is clear that much more needs to be done. James Henry estimates that tinnitus is about 40 years behind hearing loss relative to standardization of basic testing techniques.

A landmark in the history of tinnitus research was the establishment, in 1971, of the American Tinnitus Association (ATA). Founded by Jack Vernon and Charles Unice, the ATA is a major source of funding for tinnitus research, especially seed money to establish younger investigators. Since 1980 the ATA has awarded more than four million dollars in research grants focused on understanding the causes, evaluation and treatment of tinnitus.

Although tinnitus is being explored by experts in many disciplines, audiologists will undoubtedly continue to play major roles in this arena.

10

Hearing Conservation

The great artillery battles of World War I heightened awareness of the risks to the auditory system from blasts, explosions, and gunfire. But it was not until World War II, with millions of servicemen under arms, and in combat, that the problem of hearing loss from noise exposure began to be viewed as a significant health risk. It became a major concern of the Aural Rehabilitation Services at the Army's three centers at Butler, Pennsylvania, Santa Barbara, California, and Chikasaw, Oklahoma, and the Navy's center in Philadelphia. The concerns highlighted in these military programs led to a series of postwar regulatory documents; first by the newly formed U.S. Air Force in 1948, then by the Navy in 1955 and the Army in 1956. These documents not only defined noise exposure as a hazard, but set forth conditions under which hearing protection must be used, and required that personnel exposed to potentially hazardous noises be monitored eudiometrically. An important factor driving interest in hearing conservation was the high noise levels encountered after the introduction of jet aircraft into both the Air Force and the Navy in the late 1940s.

The Navy's concern for the damaging effects of noise began in earnest at the Naval School of Aviation Medicine (NSAM) in Pensacola, Florida in the early 1940s. Under the leadership of Ashton Graybiel, Director of Medical Research, NSAM carried out a systematic research program highlighting the effects of noise and flight on the auditory and vestibular systems. In addition, the school contracted, during and after the war, with Mack Steer, at Purdue University and John Black at Ohio State University for pioneering studies of speech communication issues associated with noisy environments. In this same period, the 1940s and 1950s, similar research programs were initiated by J. Donald Harris and Russell Sargeant at the Navy's submarine base at Groton, Connecticut, and by John Webster at the Navy Electronics Laboratory in San Diego. During the 1950s and 1960s, the Office of Naval Research (ONR) funded a number of university studies relating to hearing in noise and noise-induced hearing loss. Gilbert Tolhurst spearheaded much of this program. Charles Nixon, of the Bioacoustics and Biocommunications Armstrong Laboratory at Wright-Patterson Air Force Base has pointed out that the first comprehensive hearing conservation program was implemented in the military 15 years before the OSHA regulation of 1970.

Concerns about intense jet engine noise levels on the flight line and on the aircraft carrier deck led to the formation of the Committee on Hearing and Bioacoustics (CHABA) by the National Academy of Sciences—National Research Council (NAS-NRC). All

71

three services participated in CHABA along with panels of distinguished scientists drawn from the universities and from industry. Over the years a number of audiologists served on CHABA. Its initial charge was to study the biological effects of noise. In 1953 the National Research Council published its landmark report, "Biological Effects of Noise Exploratory Study (BENOX)," which summarized, for the first time in one document, the many sequelae of intense noise exposure, including aural pain, hearing loss, communication problems, psychological effects, communication problems, difficulty orienting in space, and other effects on the central nervous system.

One of the leaders in the early years of military hearing conservation was the bioacoustics research group at the Wright-Patterson Air Force base in Ohio. Henning Von Gierke, and Elizabeth Guild, in particular, were early investigators of diverse military noise environments, human tolerance limits, and hearing protective devices. While at Wright-Patterson, Guild pioneered hearing conservation well before it was mandated by either the military or civilian sectors. Later, Charles Nixon and Dan Johnson carried out a number of significant studies of adverse noise effects. The first hearing conservation data repository was established at the USAF School of Aerospace Medicine in San Antonio in 1956.

As a consequence of these studies and reports, the military services began to see the need for audiologists to design and administer hearing conservation programs. The first to do so was the Air Force. In 1957 it recruited two audiologists. The other two services soon followed; the Army acquired 11 audiologists in 1966, the Navy, 10 audiologists in 1979. One of the great dividends of these military hearing conservation programs has been the number of audiologists who, upon leaving the military, brought their knowledge and skills relative to hearing conservation to the civilian sector.

Until 1969 there was little interest in hearing conservation programs within the civilian sector. But in that year the Walsh-Healey Public Contracts Act (PCA) of 1936, which placed a number of requirements on suppliers contracting with the United States government for goods or supplies worth at least $10,000, was amended to include protection of the health of workers involved in the production of such goods or supplies.

It is often said that legal statements are among the most boring examples of prose in the English language. But the following excerpt from the 1970 amendment to the Walsh-Healey act, in one seemingly unending run-on sentence, has contributed immeasurably to the preservation of hearing in American workers:

That no part of such contract will be performed nor will any of the materials, supplies, articles, or equipment to be manufactured or furnished under said contract be manufactured or fabricated in any plants, factories, buildings, or surroundings or under working conditions which are unsanitary or hazardous or dangerous to the health and safety of employees engaged in the performance of said contract. [41 U.S.C. 35(d)]

Shortly thereafter, in 1971, Congress passed the Williams-Steiger Occupational Health Act that established the Occupational Safety and Health Administration (OSHA). This program covered all workers not already covered by the revised Walsh-Healey Public Contracts Act. Now the stage was set for the growth of hearing conservation programs within the civilian sector. But 12 more contentious years were to elapse before the OSHA published its regulatory guidelines in 1983. They established standards for maximum allowable noise environments, the time/intensity trading rule (whenever the intensity of the noise increases by 5 dB the allowable duration of exposure is shortened by a factor of 2), procedures for noise abatement (both engineering and administrative controls), and protection of the workers hearing (including both hearing protective devices and audiometric monitoring). The need for industrial hearing conservation programs was now firmly established, and many audiologists established consulting services. Audiologists who have played key roles in hearing conservation in the civilian sector include Alice Suter, David Lipscomb, Alan Feldman, William Melnick, and Donald Henderson.

In 1978 the Department of Defense (DOD), in the interest of uniformity of hearing conservation programs in all branches of the military, issued instructions mandating that all services must meet or exceed the OSHA guidelines. Finally, in 1999, all three services adopted a common computer-based test system and a common Internet-based data repository. Military audiologists who have been instrumental in implementing hearing conservation programs include David Chandler of the U.S. Army, Donald Gasaway and Ben Sierra of the U.S. Air Force, and John Page of the U.S. Navy.

Any discussion of hearing conservation in the United States must include the many contributions of Aram Glorig (Figure 10–1). In 1952 Glorig joined the American Academy of Ophthalmology and Otolaryngology's (AAOO) subcommittee on Noise of the AAOO Conservation of Hearing Committee. Here he carried out research and surveys on noise, the results of which subsequently greatly influenced the OSHA rules of 1970 and 1983. Glorig was instrumental in founding both the American Auditory Society and the International Society of Audiology. His many contributions to our understanding of the effects of noise on the auditory system

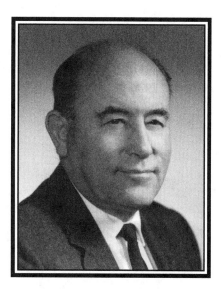

Figure 10–1. Aram Glorig.

place him among the eminent leaders in this arena.

The history of Hearing Conservation in the United States would be incomplete without citing the important contributions of Robert Dobie of the University of California at Davis. Dobie has written extensively on several aspects of hearing, hearing loss, and hearing conservation and is author of the definitive volume, *Medico-Legal Evaluation of Hearing Loss*.

Although the lion's share of interest in hearing conservation has focused on adults, there is gathering evidence that many children are at risk for noise-induced hearing loss. Principal suspects include hunting, snowmobiling, and the ubiquitous i-Pod. Yet, in spite of the established need, school-based hearing conservation programs are rare. This is one of the most important challenges facing our profession today. Although we have succeeded in screening almost all newborn babies, we have sadly neglected school-aged children whose hearing may be at risk.

SECTION III

Professional Growth

The history of any profession is intimately related to four factors: (1) its interactions with related professions, (2) the educational institutions and policies that influence the training of its members, (3) the professional organizations that provide a home for its members, and (4) the sources of research support for its scientific base. In this section, we consider how the growth of audiology has been influenced by these four factors.

11

The Medical Connection

Throughout its history, audiology has been strongly influenced by related medical specialties, particularly otolaryngology. Early pioneers included Los Angeles otologist Isaac Jones who collaborated with legendary acoustician Vernon Knudsen, head of the physics department at UCLA in the 1920s, to develop the first audiometer with bone conduction testing capability; otolaryngologist L. W. Dean, who mentored the young C. C. Bunch; otolaryngologist Walter Hughson, who collaborated with speech pathologist Harold Westlake in the development of the well-known "Hughson-Westlake" protocol for obtained a pure-tone audiometric threshold; and, of course, physiologist Hallowell Davis, whose many contributions have already been discussed.

Many long-standing and fruitful collaborations between audiologists and otolaryngologists arose from a common interest in patients with medically treatable hearing disorders. The development of the fenestration operation, by Julius Lempert in 1938, and subsequent techniques of stapes mobilization pioneered by Sam Rosen in the early 1950s, created an unusual opportunity for a mutual collaboration between otologic surgeons and audiologists in documenting and quantifying the improvement in hearing provided by surgical intervention. One example was the collaboration between Raymond Carhart,

head of the audiology program in Northwestern University's School of Speech, and George Shambaugh, chairman of the department of otolaryngology in Northwestern's School of Medicine. Shambaugh was one of the pioneers of the fenestration operation, in which a surgeon creates an opening in a semicircular canal to bypass the middle ear mechanism immobilized by otosclerosis. Throughout the decade of the 1950s, Carhart and Shambaugh jointly staffed a weekly otology/audiology clinic in which Carhart and his audiology students carried out audiologic assessments and Shambaugh and his residents carried out the medical evaluations of a small number of patients from Shambaugh's practice. Then the patients were jointly counseled by Carhart and Shambaugh. It was an excellent example of how the two disciplines could collaborate in an atmosphere of mutual respect, for the benefit of hearing-impaired persons: and, it was a teaching experience of unparalleled value to all who participated. It was this collaboration that resulted in the now famous "Carhart notch," the characteristic depression in the bone conduction threshold at 2000 Hz in persons with otosclerosis.

Another example of early collaboration between audiologists and otolaryngologists occurred at the Louisiana State University (LSU) Medical School in New Orleans. Here audiologist Charles Berlin and otolaryngologist Merv Trail collaborated on a research and clinical program of unusual productivity for over 20 years.

At the University of California at Los Angeles (UCLA), audiologist Donald Dirks collaborated, first with otolaryngologist Victor Goodhill and later with Goodhill's successor, Paul Ward, in the development of an audiologic research program of international renown.

The success of these early collaborations convinced many audiologists and otolaryngologists that they could take maximum advantage of each other's expertise by working together in the same medical department. Such collaborations continue to flourish today in many academic medical settings.

Unfortunately, the course of these interactions has not always been smooth: frictions have sometimes arisen. In his classic book, *Clinical Audiometry*, published in 1943, C. C. Bunch noted that an otologist had publicly stated that he had no confidence in audiometric tests because he had been sent three entirely different audiograms of the same patient by three different testers. Bunch suggested that a report of this sort would have been impossible if the tests had been carried out under proper conditions by trained examiners, using standardized audiometers and careful testing technique.

A particular point of contention in today's world has been the reaction of some otolaryngologists to audiology's attempts to upgrade the qualifications of its practitioners. Because a significant percentage of audiologists are employed in medical settings, and usually in departments headed by otolaryngologists, there is a persistent concern among our medical colleagues who view audiologists as valued but nonetheless

technicians, and fear that upgrading to the Au.D. degree will both increase the cost of employing audiologists and result in overqualified personnel. Periodically, they have threatened to train their own audiometric technicians to fill the roles presently played by audiologists with master's and Au.D. degrees. Indeed, they have recently developed a program known as CPOP (Certificate Program for Otolaryngology Personnel) with an initial concentration on the training of audiometric technicians. The extent to which such activities among the medical ranks will impact audiology diminishes as our field moves more and more in the direction of private practice.

In general, collaboration between audiologists and otolaryngologists historically has been most successful when the audiologist held the Ph.D. degree, and least successful when the audiologist held only a master's degree. In the former case, mutual respect was more easily achieved than in the latter case. One of the theoretical benefits of upgrading from the master's degree to the Au.D. degree was the idea that this would help to foster an atmosphere of coequality in medical settings. Whether this hope will fall victim to the financial concerns noted above only time will reveal.

In summary, the strong relationships and good will built between audiology and otolaryngology in the early years remain in force in many medical settings, certainly to the advantage of both disciplines. But as our profession matures and moves in new directions there have been, and will undoubtedly continue to be, strains and frictions between the two arenas. Hopefully, the issues underlying any conflicts will be resolved amicably so that each discipline can continue to benefit from mutual interaction.

12

Audiologic Education

The earliest educational programs devoted specifically to training in audiology were organized in the late 1940s and early 1950s. Initially, they were concentrated in the Midwest, especially at Northwestern University, the University of Iowa, and Purdue University. Within a decade, however, there was a training program at almost every other Big Ten university. Then the movement spread to the southern, western, and eastern regions of the country. By the 1990s, there were no less than 135 programs leading to the master's degree, and 50 programs leading to the Ph.D. degree in audiology.

It is important to understand how these programs developed historically. As early as the 19th century, the liberal arts departments of many universities in the United States harbored programs in speech, debate, elocution, and theater. A natural outgrowth of this emphasis on speech communication skills was the development of a subspecialty of "speech correction" for children and adults with disorders of speech production. Faculty members with a particular interest in the diagnosis and treatment of speech disorders first developed courses on speech correction, then organized outpatient clinics in which students could practice skills acquired academically. The professional home for faculty members in speech departments in those days was an organization called the National Association of Teachers of Speech (NATS). But as the specialization of speech correction continued to develop there was a gathering unrest among its promoters; they felt that their unique contributions were not being appropriately appreciated by the NATS. In 1925 they broke away from NATS and formed the American Academy of Speech Correction. Later the name was changed to the American Speech and Hearing Association (ASHA), and finally, in 1978, to the American Speech-Language-Hearing Association (but still retaining the ASHA acronym).

There was, of course, a good deal of soul searching about disloyalty to the parent organization, and well into the 1950s many prominent ASHA leaders continued to attend the NATS convention every year. But eventually the old ties were severed completely. Today, few audiologists remember the National Association of Teachers of Speech although it is still a major player in the academic world; NATS changed its name in 1946 to The Speech Association of America.

In most universities, the new specialization of speech correction continued to be housed within the traditional department of speech, but the ties that bound it grew ever weaker. Then a new actor appeared on the scene. Following the success of the World War II military auditory rehabilitation programs, the academic people who had been involved in these centers returned to their university posts anxious to continue the thrust by adding courses in hearing testing, amplification, and aural rehabilitation to the curricula of their departments. At Northwestern University, where speech was an entire school rather than a program within a department of liberal arts, this expansion was easily achieved and the Northwestern program was an early leader in the development of a specifically audiologic curriculum. Indeed, the first Ph.D. degree in audiology was awarded by the Northwestern program in 1946 to John Keys who went on to establish a successful program at the Oklahoma University Medical Center.

Not unexpectedly, the development of audiology programs tended to follow the model already developed in the speech correction arena. In this model, there was a clear hierarchy. At the undergraduate level students were prepared to function as special education teachers—to work directly with children and adults with speech disorders, usually in the public schools. Until very recently a bachelor's degree sufficed for this role. At the graduate level students were trained to function as teachers and supervisors of undergraduate students, usually in university clinic settings. Here, the Ph.D. degree was virtually required.

As audiology programs developed they tended to follow this same model but with one exception: the workers in the field, basically audiometrists, were trained at the master's degree level. At the teacher/supervisor level, however, the Ph.D. was still the required degree. For many years, a principal venue of employment for master's degree audiologists was the hospital clinic or physicians office. Here, they functioned in a role that is best described as "doctor's helper," providing a second tier, or laboratory, service. Holders of the Ph.D. degree continued to play the role of teacher, mentor, and supervisor, usually in the university setting.

In 1979, however, a single event altered audiologic reality. ASHA declared that it was no longer unethical to dispense hearing aids. For the first time, the possibility of meaningful private practice loomed on the horizon. Instead of a second-tier role as adviser and helper to other professionals, the audiologist could function as a first-tier, point of entry into the health care system.

The Au.D. Degree

At this point a few farsighted individuals, led by David Goldstein (Figure 12–1) of Purdue University, urged a major reform in audiologic education; upgrading from the master's degree level of training to a doctoral level, insisting that such a change was essential to the emergence of a truly independent health care profession. In spite of considerable opposition, they persevered and succeeded in planting the seeds from which the audiologic doctor's degree, the Au.D., has grown and flourished.

Since the initiation of the first Au.D. degree program, at the Baylor College of Medicine in Houston in 1992, other Au.D. programs have been developed at 73 institutions across the country. Predictably, the

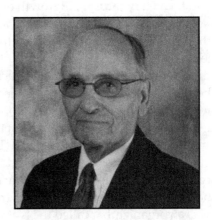

Figure 12–1. David Goldstein.

growth of Au.D. programs has forced a corresponding decline in the number of master's degree programs. It is too early to tell whether the number of Ph.D. degree programs will suffer a similar decline. The Au.D. degree is one of the cornerstones supporting the ultimate and inevitable development of audiology as a truly independent health care profession.

Practice Management

Private practioners have long lamented the lack of educational courses aimed at the essentials of business practice. They have argued that, even at the doctoral level, graduates are usually ill prepared to address the business issues relating to the management of a private practice. But this problem is now being aggressively addressed by a number of individuals; foremost among them has been Holly Hosford-Dunn (Figure 12–2) who has written extensively on practice management in audiology. Other important contributions in the areas of outcome measures, marketing principles, audiology practice design, management of human resources, business plans,

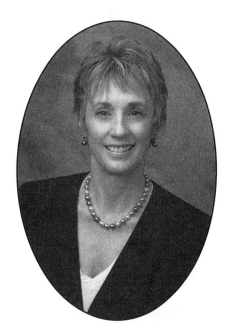

Figure 12–2. Holly Hosford-Dunn. (Courtesy of Jon Wolf/Tucson, AZ.)

accounting, financial management, and other aspects of practice management have been made by Harvey Abrams, Darcy Benson, Theresa Chisolm, Teresa Clark, Barry Freeman, Gail Gudmundsen, Gyl Kasewurm, Paul Pessis, Marjorie Skafte, Wayne Staab, Ian Windmill, and David Zapala.

13

Professional Organizations

During the past half century audiologists have found a professional home in five different organizations; the American Speech, Language, Hearing Association (ASHA), the Academy of Rehabilitative Audiology (ARA), the American Auditory Society (AAS), The Academy of Doctors of Audiology (ADA), and the American Academy of Audiology (AAA). There are, to be sure, a number of other organizations catering to one or more specialized interests, but these five have had by far the greatest influence on the growth of the profession. Many audiologists are also members of international groups like the Educational Audiology Association and the International Society of Audiology; but international groups are beyond the scope of this book.

The American Speech-Language-Hearing Association (ASHA)

ASHA was formed in 1925 as the American Academy of Speech Correction (AASC). During its first two decades it was largely an organization of speech scientists and speech therapists. Indeed, most of the early leaders of audiology came from the AASC ranks. At the end of World War II, those members who had been involved in the wartime aural rehabilitation programs, returned to their prewar home, the AASC. Before long, however, they were agitating for recognition of the new specialty of audiology within their traditional professional home. Accordingly, the AASC soon changed its name to the American Speech and Hearing Association (ASHA), then in 1978 to its present name, the American Speech-Language-Hearing Association (but retaining the acronym ASHA).

Throughout the 1950s and 1960s, ASHA was the sole professional home for audiologists. Under the leadership of Executive Secretary Kenneth O. Johnson, and many respected members of the academic community, ASHA took the important step of establishing a certification program designed to guarantee minimal standards of preparation and competence of audiologists providing clinical services. Then, in the 1970s and 1980s, as more and more states created licensing statutes, ASHA certification, as the only viable guarantor of competence, became the *sine qua non* of qualification for licensing. During those years, as audiology sought to establish and strengthen its professional image, ASHA's role in certification and licensing was generally viewed in a positive light by most audiologists. But ASHA made one decision that several viewed as a tactical error. They tied ASHA certification to ASHA membership, which meant, in effect, that state licensing required audiologists to maintain ASHA membership. In time this came to be resented by many influential audiologists, who argued that in no other profession was the ability to practice in a state through licensure tied to membership in a professional organization. Subsequent actions by ASHA, including early opposition to the Au.D. degree, reluctance to create standards specifically for the Au.D., and unwillingness to share the Au.D. accreditation process with other organizations, further alienated many audiologists. To its credit, however, in recent years, ASHA seems to have made a sincere effort to give greater recognition and status to its remaining audiology members in its publications and at its conventions. It has also lobbied the federal government for many issues of concern to audiologists.

The Academy of Rehabilitative Audiology (ARA)

The seeds of discontent with ASHA as the professional home for audiologists had already begun to grow in the 1960s with the establishment of the Academy of Rehabilitative Audiology. Following the 1964 ASHA convention in San Francisco, a group of audiologists, John O'Neill, Herbert Oyer, Jack Rosen, and Mary Rose Costello met to address the concern that the rehabilitative aspects of audiology were not being adequately served by ASHA. They concluded that the subspecialty of rehabilitation audiology needed its own professional home in order to:

1. stimulate scientific research in the area of rehabilitation of auditorily handicapped children and adults and

2. provide a forum for the exchange of information and viewpoints important to rehabilitative audiology.

A group of leaders in aural rehabilitation were invited to a meeting in 1965 to establish the academy. The original founders were: Charlotte Avery, Francis X. Blair, Mary Rose Costello, D. Robert Frisina, Richard Krug, Freeman McConnell, June Miller, John O'Neill, Herbert Oyer, L. Deno Reed, and Jack Rosen.

The ARA was formally launched in 1966 at a meeting at Gallaudet College (now Gallaudet University). It now hosts a summer institute each year, and has published, since 1967, the *Journal of the Academy of Rehabilitative Audiology*. ARA presently has approximately 200 members.

Other audiologists have had similar complaints, that specialized interests were not given sufficient recognition by ASHA. In 1958, for example, a plan to create special interest groups within ASHA was presented to the Executive Council by an audiologist. It met with no success. The counter argument was that any such move was divisive and threatened the stability of the organization. It was not until many years later that the special interest group concept was finally, albeit reluctantly, accepted by ASHA.

A further source of discontent among audiologists was the ASHA Code of Ethics with respect to the dispensation of hearing aids; dispensing was declared to be unethical and grounds for loss of membership. This was viewed by many as a major stumbling block toward the establishment of private practice, a development that many felt was essential if audiology was to become an independent health care profession. As early as 1974, the ARA had argued that the quality of professional services, not the economic objections raised by ASHA, should be the basis on which the decision to dispense aids should be based.

The Academy of Doctors of Audiology (ADA)

In 1977 a group of audiologists particularly interested in the dispensing of hearing aids met in Colorado Springs, Colorado to launch the Academy of Dispensing Audiologists (ADA). Founding members included Leo Doerfler, John Maher, John Balko, Norman Carmel, Chauncey Hewitt, Michael Pollack, Roy Rowland, and Anthony Tsappis. The first meeting of the new group was held in San Francisco late in 1978 and elected Leo Doerfler as its first president. From its inception ADA has been an organization devoted to the advancement of autonomous audiology private practice and practitioner excellence. It has been particularly effective in its support of the Au.D. concept and of Au.D. educational programs. ADA now numbers approximately 800 members. Recently, the organization has changed its name to the "Academy of Doctors of Audiology," and has set as its goal, in its new vision statement, increasing the percentage of audiologists in private practice from its present 20% to 80%.

The American Auditory Society (AAS)

The American Auditory Society, originally the American Audiology Society, was founded in 1972. The organizational meeting, called by Aram Glorig, was held in Dallas, Texas. Founding members included William Carver, Peter Dallos, Mike Dennis, Marion Downs, Alan Goodman, Bruce Graham, Donnell Johns, Fernando Kirchner, Paula Menyuk, Ralph Naunton, Harris Pomerantz, Louis Ranney, Ross Roeser, Roy Rowland, Blair Simmons, Jeanne Smith, Jurgen Tonndorf, and Laura Wilber. Founders agreed that the purpose of AAS was to unite the various disciplines involved in "hearing." There was a felt need for a "nonpolitical" organization where clinicians and researchers in audiology, otolaryngology, and the engineering/industry sector could meet to exchange findings and new ideas.

At the first official meeting, in Dallas in 1973, Aram Glorig was elected president and the principle was established that AAS meetings would coincide with the annual meetings of three different professional groups, the American Speech and Hearing Association (ASHA), the American Academy of Otolaryngology (AAO), and the Acoustical Society of America (ASA). For various reasons, this idea didn't work out too well. Finally, in 1996, the AAS decided to organize its own meeting independently of other groups. Since then it has been held in the spring of each year in the Phoenix, Arizona area, with considerable success. A popular feature of its annual meeting is the Carhart Memorial Lecture, given each year since 1976 by outstanding leaders representative of the multidisciplinary nature of the membership. In 1977 the organization changed to its present name, The American Auditory Society.

In 1975 the AAS published the first issue of its official scientific publication, the *Journal of the American Audiology Society*, with J. Donald Harris as editor-in-chief. In 1980 the name of the journal was changed to *Ear and Hearing* Within the past three decades, *Ear and Hearing* has become a highly respected publication.

The goal of AAS has always been to provide a multidisciplinary venue in which audiologists, otolaryngologists, dispensers, psychoacousticians, and engineers may meet and share a formal platform for the interchange of information. AAS has approximately 2500 members, about 80% of whom are audiologists.

The American Academy of Audiology (AAA)

The American Academy of Audiology was founded in 1988 in response to a rising sense that, in spite of the existing organizations, audiologists as a whole, still lacked their own unique professional home. The idea of forming an organization of, by, and for audiologists first took root at the 1987 ASHA convention in New Orleans. Rick Talbot had organized a session in which he asked five individuals, Jay Hall, Lucille Beck, George Osborne, Charles Berlin, and James Jerger, to speculate on the future of audiology. In Jerger's talk he suggested that perhaps it was time for audiologists to form their own professional organization. The response from the audience shocked everyone. There was such a roar of approval for the idea that Jerger started to think seriously about the feasibility of such a move. Although he had long felt that audiology needed more autonomy, he was not sure how many audiologists shared this view. Moreover, the obstacles to a move toward greater independence had always seemed insurmountable. Back in Houston Jerger talked the idea over with colleague and good friend, Brad Stach. They agreed that it was something they at least ought to try to do.

The actual founding of the Academy proved to be considerably less difficult than expected. Stach and Jerger put together a list of 35 individuals whom they thought might be interested in supporting the concept of a new organization. Then they wrote to each person inviting him/her to come to Houston for a two-day meeting to discuss the idea of forming our own professional organization. Almost everyone who was invited came to the meeting. The individuals who attended this initial meeting, the founders of the academy, are as follows:

Lucille Beck, Fred Bess, Tomi Browne, David Citron, Michael Dennis, Leo Doerfler, David Goldstein, James Hall III, Maureen Hannley, Robert Harrison, Linda Hood, John Jacobson, James Jerger, Susan Jerger, Robert Keith, Paul Kileny, Vernon Larson, H. Gus Mueller, Frank Musiek, Jerry Northern, Wayne Olsen, George Osborne, Anita Pikus, Ross Roeser, Roger Ruth, Daniel Schwartz, Brad Stach, Laszlo Stein, Roy Sullivan, Richard Talbott, Laura Wilber, and Don Worthington.

The meeting was certainly interesting. After the first morning, people were shaking their heads in dismay, wondering whether this group would ever be able to agree on anything. But by the end of the second day, there was a fairly good consensus that the effort at least ought to be made.

The first year of the Academy's existence, 1988, was an uncertain time. The founders were not at all sure that their efforts would succeed. They knew what they wanted to do and where they wanted to go, but recognized with some trepidation the formidable forces arrayed against them. The primary concern was, of course, the ASHA. It already counted, at that time, more than 8000 audiologists among its roughly 60,000 members, and was not disposed to view this defection in a collegial manner. It was not certain how many of these individuals would be attracted to a new organization.

The first national office was set up at the Baylor College of Medicine in Houston. Brad Stach (Figure 13–1), who then supervised Baylor's Audiology Service at the Methodist Hospital in Houston, was the first secretary-treasurer of the new organization. He was instrumental in bringing the concept of a new organization to concrete reality. He set up the original organizational structure, implemented the solicitation of new members, corresponded with existing members, and generally kept the ship on course.

Gus Mueller (Figure 13–2), as chair of the first membership committee, was faced

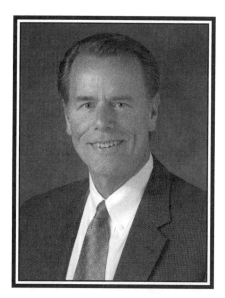

Figure 13–1. Brad Stach. (Courtesy of Riva Sayegh, Henry Ford Hospital.)

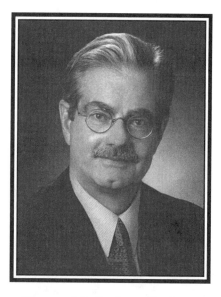

Figure 13–3. Jerry Northern.

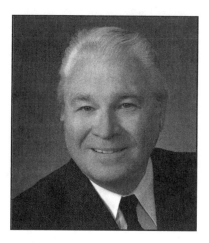

Figure 13–2. Gus Mueller.

with the truly difficult task of applying what were sometimes vague and abstract definitions of membership qualifications to the credentials of actual applicants. During that first year, the membership climbed to more than 1500 audiologists, a far higher figure than anyone had imagined possible in so short a time. By June of 1989, membership had reached 2000.

Encouraged by this rapid growth the academy set in motion the creation of the two main academy publications, *Audiology Today* and the *Journal of the American Academy of Audiology*. During that first year, *Audiology Today* was created as a desktop publishing venture of the national office under the creative direction of Terrey Oliver Penn. Subsequent years have seen the production raised to a more polished level by former editors John Jacobson and Jerry Northern (Figure 13–3).

The highlight of 1989 was the memorable first annual convention held at Kiawah Island, South Carolina. Verne Larson chose the site; president-elect Fred Bess organized the program and supervised virtually every detail of its execution. The theme was "Audiology— A New Beginning." It was a resounding success. From that point on, a bright future lay ahead of us, and there was no looking back. The American Academy of Audiology now includes more than 11,000 members and has become the professional home for audiologists in the United States.

14

Research Support for Audiology

Audiologic research has been supported by a number of organizations over the past six decades. Federal government sources have included the National Institutes of Health, the U.S. Department of Education, the Department of Defense, the Office of Naval Research, the U.S. Army, the U.S. Air Force, the Vocational Rehabilitation Administration, the National Science Foundation, and the Department of Veterans Affairs. Some of these agencies have changed names over the years, and some are defunct, but federal support has been continuous. The principal nongovernmental sources of support have been the Deafness Research Foundation and a number of smaller foundations supporting research in specifically targeted areas.

By far the single most important source of research support has been the National Institutes of Health (NIH). Support began in the 1950 with the creation of the National Institute on Neurological Diseases and Blindness (NINDB). Raymond Carhart, of Northwestern University, Wendell Johnson, of the University of Iowa, and William Hardy, of the Johns Hopkins University, were early advisors to the Institute on how it might support research in the speech and hearing areas. The creation of NINDB was followed rapidly by establishment of the National Institute of Child Health and Human Development (NICHD) in 1963 and the National

Institute on Aging (NIA) in 1974. After creation of the National Eye Institute, in 1968, the name of the original NINDB was changed to the National Institute on Neurological Diseases and Stroke. In 1975 that name was changed, again, to the National Institute of Neurological and Communicative Disorders and Stroke (NINCDS), the first recognition of the speech and hearing specialties in the name of an Institute. Finally, in 1988, thanks to the efforts of many professionals in the speech, hearing, and deafness fields, and a number of key nonprofessionals, the National Institute on Deafness and other Communicative Disorders (NIDCD) was formed under the authority of Public Law 100-553. Here, for the first time in the history of the National Institutes of Health, there was a separate Institute devoted exclusively to "disorders of hearing and other communicative processes including diseases affecting hearing, balance, voice, speech, language, taste, and smell."

Over the years, a number of audiologists and hearing scientists have served on the study sections that review NIH grant applications. Some who have recently served in this all important role for the profession include Judy Dubno, Marjorie Leek, Pat Stelmachowicz, Michael Dorman, Sandra Gordon-Salant, Michael Gorga, Susan Jerger, Laurie Eisenberg, Joseph Hall, Brenda Ryals, Brenda Lonsbury-Martin, and Paul Kileny.

Throughout this long period of NIH growth, fragmentation, reformation, and re-naming, speech and hearing scientists have enjoyed a long history of research support, principally from NIDCD and its antecedents, but also from the NICHD, and from NIA. It is certainly the case that this support, sustained for so many years, has been one of the major sources of strength for our profession.

15

Looking Back

What lessons can we take away from this brief historical review of a profession's growth? Perhaps one of the most important is the inevitability of fragmentation. Over the past half century, audiology has seen the development of specializations that have tended to splinter off into new organizations. Indeed, audiology itself splintered off from the parent field of speech correction. And speech correction splintered off from teachers of speech. Whenever this happens there is always grim talk of disloyalty, and of the need to preserve the unity of the original group, but, as we have seen, fragmentation goes on in spite of prophets of doom and disaster. It is the natural consequence of growth. Like the tide it cannot be easily held back. We have seen how speech correctionists splintered off from teachers of speech (ASHA), how audiologists broke away from speech-language pathologists (AAA), and how audiologists, themselves, have formed separate organizations recognizing the spe-

cial interests of aural rehabilitationists (ARA), hearing aid dispensers (ADA), and multidisciplinary auditory researchers (AAS). Professional maturity will perhaps be reached when all organizations have learned to work together for the common good rather than anguishing over fragmentation and sparring with each other over turf and influence.

Although this brief review has traced six distinct paths in which the profession has developed over the past half century, it is interesting to observe the degree to which these paths have interacted. We see the fruits of progress in the diagnostic path reflected in the development of APD and tinnitus testing, the impact of advances in electroacoustics and electrophysiology on universal screening procedures, the influence of cochlear implant advances on auditory training, and the influences of all paths on intervention with amplification. These are, I believe, hallmarks of a robust and growing profession with a remarkable history.

Sources and Suggested Readings

Abrams, H., & Hnath-Chisolm. (2000). Outcome measures: The audiologic difference. In H. Hosford-Dunn, R. Roeser, & M. Valente (Eds.), *Audiology practice management*. New York: Thieme.

Arnst, D., & Katz, J. (Eds.). (1982). *Central auditory assessment: The SSW test*. San Diego, CA: College-Hill Press.

ASHA Task Force on Central Auditory Processing Consensus Development. (1996). Central auditory processing: current status of research and implications for clinical practice. *American Journal of Audiology, 5*, 41–54.

Bellis, T. (1996). *Assessment and management of central auditory processing disorders in the educational setting: From science to practice*. San Diego, CA: Singular.

Berger, K. W. (1976). Genealogy of the words "audiology" and "audiologist." *Journal of the American Audiology Society, 2*, 38–44.

Bergman, M. (2001). American wartime military audiology. *Audiology Today* (Monograph #1), pp. 1–24.

Berlin, C., Lowe, S., Thompson, L., & Cullen, J. (1968). The construction and perception of simultaneous messages. *ASHA, 10*, 397.

Bocca, E., Calearo, C., Cassinari, V., & Migliavacca, F. (1955). Testing "cortical" hearing in temporal lobe tumors. *Acta Otolaryngologica, 45*, 289–304.

Bonfils, P., Avan, P., Francois, M., Marie, P., Trotoux, J., & Narcy, P. (1990). Clinical significance of otoacoustic emissions: A perspective. *Ear and Hearing, 11*, 155–158.

Brackett, D., Maxon, A., & Blackwell, P. (1993). Intervention issues created by successful universal newborn hearing screening. *Seminars in Hearing, 14*, 88–104.

Broadbent, D. (1958). *Perception and communication*. New York: Macmillan.

Brownell, W. E. (1990). Outer hair cell electromotility and otoacoustic emissions. *Ear and Hearing, 11*(2), 82–92.

Bryden, M. (1963). Ear preference in auditory perception. *Journal of Experimental Psycholology, 16*, 291–299.

Bunch, C. (1941). The development of the audiometer. *Laryngoscope, 52*, 1100–1118.

Bunch, C. (1943). *Clinical audiometry*. St. Louis, MO: Mosby.

Bureau of Labor Statistics, U. S. Deptartment of Labor. (2008). *Occupational outlook handbook, audiologists*. Retrieved January 06, 2008.

Cacace, A., & McFarland, D. (1998). Central auditory processing disorder in school-aged children: A critical review. *Journal of Speech, Language and Hearing Research, 41*, 355–373.

Calearo, C., & Lazzaroni, A. (1957). Speech intelligibility in relation to the speed of the message. *Laryngoscope, 67*, 410–419.

Canfield, N. (1949). Audiology: *The science of hearing*. Springfield, IL: Charles C. Thomas.

Carhart, R. (1946). Tests for the selection of hearing aids. *Laryngoscope, 56*, 780–794.

Compton, C. (2002). Assistive technology for the enhancement of receptive communication. In J. A. P. McCarthy (Ed.), *Rehabilitation audiology*. Baltimore: Williams & Wilkins.

Cox, R., & Alexander, G. (1995). The abbreviated profile of hearing aid benefit. *Ear and Hearing, 16*, 176–186.

Cox, R., & Alexander, G. (1999). Measuring satisfaction with amplification in daily life: SADL. *Ear and Hearing, 20*, 306–320.

Cox, R., & Alexander, C. (2002). The International Outcome Inventory for Hearing Aids (IOI-HA):

psychometric properties of the English version. *International Journal of Audiology, 41*, 30–35.

Davidson, R., & Hugdahl, K. (Eds.). (1998). *Brain asymmetry*. Cambridge, MA: MIT Press.

Davis, H. (Ed.). (1947). *Hearing and deafness: A guide for laymen*. New York: Murray Hill Books.

Davis, H. (1965). Slow cortical responses evoked by acoustic stimuli. *Acta Otolaryngologica, 59*, 179–185.

Dix, M., Hallpike, C., & Hood, J. (1948). Observations upon the loudness recruitment phenomenon with especial reference to the differential diagnosis of disorders of the internal ear and VIII nerve. *Proceedings of the Royal Society of Medicine, 41*, 516–526.

Downs, M. (1990). Twentieth century pediatric audiology: Prologue to the 21st. *Seminars in Hearing, 11*, 408–411.

Egan, J. (1948). Articulation testing methods. *Laryngoscope, 58*, 955–991.

Eisenberg, L. (2007). Current state of knowledge: speech recognition and production in children with hearing impairment. *Ear and Hearing, 28*, 766–772.

Feldmann, H. (1970). *A history of audiology: A comprehensive report and bibliography from the earliest beginnings to the present*. Chicago: Beltone Institute for Hearing Research.

Ferre, J. (2006). Management strategies for APD. In T. Parthasarathy (Ed.), *An introduction to auditory processing disorders in children* (pp. 161–185). Mahwah, NJ: Lawrence Erlbaum Associates.

Gatehouse, S. (1990). Determinants of self-reported disability in older subjects. *Ear and Hearing, 11*(5, Suppl.), 57S–65S.

Gatehouse, S. (1991). The contribution of central auditory factors to auditory disability. *Acta Otolaryngololologica, 476*(Suppl.), 182–188.

Glorig, A., Quiggle, R., Wheeler, D., & Grings, W. (1956). Determination of the normal hearing reference zero. *Journal of the Acoustical Society of America, 28*, 1110–1113.

Glorig, A., Wheeler, D., Quiggle, R., Grings, W., & Summerfield, A. (1957). 1954 Wisconsin state fair hearing survey. *American Academy of Ophthalmology and Otolaryngology*, pp. 3–111.

Goldstein, R., & Rodman, L. (1967). Early components of averaged evoked responses to rapidly repeated auditory stimuli. *Journal of Speech and Hearing Research, 10*, 697–705.

Greisen, O., & Rasmussen, P. (1970). Stapedius muscle reflexes and oto-neurological examinations in brain-stem tumors. *Acta Otolaryngologica, 70*, 365–378.

Hall, J. (2007). *New handbook of auditory evoked responses*. Boston: Allyn & Bacon.

Harford, E. (1980). The use of a miniature microphone in the ear canal for the verification of hearing aid performance. *Ear and Hearing, 1*, 329–337.

Hawkins, D., & Yacullo, W. (1984). Signal-to-noise ratio advantage of binaural hearing aids and directional microphones under different levels of reverberation. *Journal of Speech and Hearing Disorders, 49*(3), 278–286.

Hosford-Dunn, H., Roeser, R., & Valente, M. (2000). What is practice management? In H. Hosford-Dunn, R. Roeser, & M. Valente (Eds.), *Audiology practice management*. New York: Thieme.

Hugdahl, K. (Ed.). (1988). *Handbook of dichotic listening: Theory, methods and research*. New York: Wiley.

Jepsen, O. (1963). Middle ear muscle reflexes in man. In J. Jerger (Ed.), *Modern developments in audiology*. New York: Academic Press.

Jerger, J. (1960). Audiological manifestations of lesions in the auditory nervous system. *Laryngoscope, 70*, 417–425.

Jerger, J. (1970). Clinical experience with impedance audiometry. *Archives of Otolaryngology, 92*, 311–324.

Jerger, J. (1973). *Modern developments in audiology* (2nd ed.). New York: Academic Press.

Jerger, J. (1975). Diagnostic use of impedance measures. In J. Jerger (Ed.), *Handbook of clinical impedance audiometry*. New York: American Electromedics.

Jerger, J. (2008). A brief history of audiology in the United States. In S. Kramer (Ed.), *Audiology: Science to practice* (pp. 333–344). San Diego, CA: Plural.

Jerger, J. (2008). The concept of auditory processing disorder—a brief history. In A. Cacace & D. McFarland (Eds.), *Current controversies in central auditory processing disorder (CAPD)*. San Diego, CA: Plural.

Jerger, J., & Jerger, S. (1975). Clinical validity of central auditory tests. *Scandinavian Audioliology, 4,* 147–163.

Jerger, J., Speaks, C., & Trammel, J. (1968). A new approach to speech audiometry. *Journal of Speech and Hearing Disorders, 33,* 318–327.

Jerger, S. (1983). Speech audiometry. In J. Jerger (Ed.), *Pediatric audiometry* (pp. 71–93). San Diego, CA: College-Hill Press.

Jerger, S., & Jerger, J. (1981). *Auditory disorders: A manual for clinical evaluation.* Boston: Little, Brown and Company.

Jerger, S., Jerger, J., & Abrams, S. (1983). Speech audiometry in the young child. *Ear and Hearing, 4,* 56–66.

Jewett, D., & Williston, J. (1971). Auditory evoked far fields averaged from the scalp of humans. *Brain, 94,* 681–696.

Jirsa, R., & Clontz, K. (1990). Long latency auditory event related potentials from children with auditory processing disorders. *Ear and Hearing, 11,* 222–232.

Jongen, M., Smulders, F., & Heiden, J. V. D. (2007). Lateralized ERP components related to spatial orienting: Discriminating the direction of attention from processing sensory aspects of the cue. *Psychophysiology, 44,* 968–986.

Katz, J. (1977). The staggered spondaic word test. In R. Keith (Ed.), *Central auditory dysfunction.* New York: Grune & Stratton.

Keith, R. (2000). *SCAN-C: test for auditory processing disorders in children-revised.* San Antonio, TX: Psychological Corporation.

Kemp, D. (1978). Stimulated acoustic emissions from the human auditory system. *Journal of the Acoustical Society of America, 64,* 1386–1391.

Kimura, D. (1961). Some effects of temporal lobe damage on auditory perception. *Canadian Journal of Psychology, 15,* 157–165.

Kimura, D. (1967). Functional asymmetry of the brain in dichotic listening. *Cortex, 3,* 163–178.

Knudsen, V. (1939). An ear to the future. *Journal of the Acoustical Society of America, 11,* 29–36.

Kricos, P., & Holmes, A. (2007). From ear to there: A historical perspective on auditory training. *Seminars in Hearing, 28,* 89–98.

Kutas, M., & Hillyard, S. A. (1980). Reading senseless sentences: Brain potentials reflect semantic incongruity. *Science, 207,* 203–205.

Langguth, B., Hajak, G., Cacace, A., & Moller, A. (Eds.). (2007). *Tinnitus: Pathophysiology and treatment* (Progress in brain research series, Vol. 166). Amsterdam: Elsevier.

Levitt, H. (1971). Transformed up-down methods in psychoacoustics. *Journal of the Acoustical Society of America, 49,* 467–477.

Liden, G. (1969). The scope and application of current audiometric tests. *Journal of Laryngology and Otology, 83,* 507–520.

Lonsbury-Martin, B. L., & Martin, G. K. (1990). The clinical utility of distortion-product otoacoustic emissions. *Ear and Hearing, 11,* 144–154.

Lutman, M., Brown, E., & Coles, R. (1987). Self-reported disability and handicap in the population in relation to pure-tone threshold, age, sex and type of hearing loss. *British Journal of Audiology, 21,* 45–58.

Matzker, J. (1959). Two methods for the assessment of central auditory functions in cases of brain disease. *Annals of Otology, Rhinolology and Laryngology, 68,* 1185–1197.

McFarland, D., & Cacace, A. (1995). Modality specificity as a criterion for diagnosing central auditory processing disorders. *Audiology, 36,* 249–260.

McFarland, D., & Cacace, A. (2006). Current controversies in CAPD: from Procrustes bed to Pandora's box. In T. Parthasarathy (Ed.), *An introduction to auditory processing disorders in children* (pp. 247–263). Mahwah, NJ: Lawrence Erlbaum Associates.

Medwetsky, L. (2006). Spoken language processing: A convergent approach to conceptualizing (central) auditory processing. *ASHA Leader Online, 11,* 6–7, 30–31, 33.

Merzenich, M., Jenkins, W., Johnston, P., Schreiner, C., Miller, S., & Tallal, P. (1996). Temporal processing deficits of language-learning impaired children ameliorated by training. *Science, 271,* 77–81.

Milner, B. (1962). Laterality effects in audition. In V. Mountcastle (Ed.), *Interhemispheric relations and cerebral dominance* (pp. 177–195). Baltimore: The Johns Hopkins Press.

Moeller, M. P., Tomblin, J., Yoshinaga-Itano, C., Connor, C., & Jerger, S. (2007). Current state of knowledge: Language and literacy of children with hearing impairment. *Ear and Hearing, 28,* 740–753.

Moller, A. (1958). Intra-aural muscle contraction in man, examined by measuring acoustic impedance of the ear. *Laryngoscope, 68,* 48–62.

Moore, D. (2006). Auditory processing disorder (APD): Definition, diagnosis, neural basis, and intervention. *Audiological Medicine, 4,* 4–11.

Mueller, H., & Hall, J. (1998). *Audiologists' desk reference* (Vols. I and II). San Diego, CA: Singular.

Musiek, F., Baran, J., & Pinheiro, M. (1994). *Neuroaudiology case studies.* San Diego, CA: Singular.

Musiek, F., & Pinheiro, M. (1985). Dichotic speech tests in the detection of central auditory dysfunction. In M. Pinheiro & F. Musiek (Eds.), *Assessment of central auditory dysfunction: Foundations and clinical correlates* (pp. 201–219). Baltimore: Williams & Wilkins.

Myklebust, H. (1954). *Auditory disorders in children.* New York: Grune & Stratton.

Näätänen, R., & Kraus, N. (1995). Mismatch negativity as an index of central auditory function. *Ear and Hearing, 16,* 1–146.

Nabelek, A. (2005). Acceptance of background noise may be key to successful fitting. *Hearing Journal, 59,* 10–15.

Newman, C., Jacobson, G., Hug, G., Weinstein, B., & Malinoff, R. (1991). Practical method for quantifying hearing aid benefit in older adults. *Journal of the American Academy of Audiology, 2,* 70–75.

Newman, C., & Weinstein, B. (1988). The Hearing Handicap Inventory for the Elderly as a measure of hearing aid benefit. *Ear and Hearing, 9,* 85–85.

Noble, W. (1978). *Assessment of impaired hearing—A critique and a new method.* New York: Academic Press.

Noffsinger, D., & Kurdziel, S. (1979). Assessment of central auditory lesions. In W. Rintleman (Ed.), *Hearing assessment* (pp. 351–377). Baltimore: University Park Press.

Northern, J., & Downs, M. (1978). *Hearing in children* (2nd ed.). Baltimore: Williams & Wilkins.

Palmer, C. (2007). A brief history of hearing aids. *Bulletin of the New Zealand Audiological Society, 17,* 13–34.

Phillips, D. (1999). Auditory gap detection, perceptual channels, and temporal resolution in speech perception. *Journal of the American Academy of Audiology, 10,* 343–354.

Picton, T., Stapells, D., Perrault, N., Baribeau-Braun, J., & Stuss, D. (1984). Human event-related potentials: Current perspectives. In R. Nodar & C. Barber (Eds.), *Evoked potentials II: The Second International Evoked Potentials Symposium* (pp. 3–16). Boston: Butterworth.

Pinheiro, M. (1977). Tests of central auditory function in children with learning disabilities. In R. Keith (Ed.), *Central auditory dysfunction.* New York: Grune & Stratton.

Probst, R. (1990). Otoacoustic emissions: An overview. *Advances in Oto-Rhino-Laryngology, 44,* 1–91.

Rees, N. (1973). Auditory processing factors in language disorders: The view from Procrustes' bed. *Journal of Speech and Hearing Research, 38,* 304–315.

Rees, N. (1981). Saying more than we know: Is auditory processing disorder a meaningful concept. In R. Keith (Ed.), *Central auditory and language disorders in children* (pp. 94–120). San Diego, CA: College-Hill Press.

Rosen, S., Bergman, M., Plester, D., El-Mofty, A., & Satti, M. (1962). Presbycusis study of a relatively noise-free population in the Sudan. *Annals of Otology, Rhinology and Otolaryngology, 71,* 727–743.

Sharma, A., Kraus, N., McGee, T., & Nicol, T. (1997). Developmental changes in P1 and N1 central auditory responses elicited by consonant-vowel syllables. *EEG and Clinical Neurophysiology, 104,* 540–545.

Silman, S., & Silverman, C. (1991). *Auditory diagnosis: Principles and applications.* San Diego, CA: Academic Press.

Silman, S., Silverman, C., & Emmer, M. (2000). Central auditory processing disorders and reduced motivation: Three case studies. *Journal of the American Academy of Audiology, 11,* 57–63.

Skalbeck, G. (1984). The Academy of Rehabilitative Audiology: 1966–1976. *Journal of the Academy of Rehabitative Audiology, 17,* 16–58.

Sloan, C. (1980). Auditory processing disorders and language development. In P. Levinson & C. Sloan (Eds.), *Auditory processing and language:*

Clinical and research perspectives (pp. 101–116). New York: Grune & Stratton.

Sparks, R., & Geschwind, N. (1968). Dichotic listening in man after section of neocortical commissures. *Cortex, 4,* 3–16.

Speaks, C., & Jerger, J. (1965). Method for measurement of speech identification. *Journal of Speech and Hearing Research, 8,* 185–194.

Strauss, A., & Lehtinen, L. (1947). *Psychpathology and education of the brain-injured child.* New York: Grune & Stratton.

Sutton, S., Braren, M., Zubin, J., & John, E. (1965). Evoked potential correlates of stimulus uncertainty. *Science, 150,* 1187–1188.

Tallal, P. (1980). Language disabilities in children: A perceptual or linguistic deficit? *Journal of Pediatric Psychology, 5,* 127–140.

Tallal, P., Miller, S., Bedi, G., Byma, G., Wang, X., Nagarajan, S., et al. (1996). Language comprehension in language-learning impaired children improved with acoustically modified speech. *Science, 271,* 81–84.

Watson, L., & Tolan, T. (1949). *Hearing tests and hearing instruments.* Baltimore: Williams & Wilkins.

Weinstein, B., & Ventry, I. (1983). Audiometric correlates of the Hearing Handicap Inventory for the Elderly. *Journal of Speech and Hearing Disorders, 48,* 379–383.

Willeford, J. (1977). Assessing central auditory behavior in children: A test battery approach. In R. Keith (Ed.), *Central auditory dysfunction* (pp. 43–72). New York: Grune & Stratton.

Wingfield, A., & Tun, P. (2001). Spoken language comprehension in older adults: Interactions between sensory and cognitive changes in normal aging. *Seminars in Hearing, 22,* 287–301.

Woodcock, R., McGrew, K., & Mather, N. (2001). *Woodcock-Johnson III Tests of Cognitive Abilities.* Itasca, IL: Riverside.

Index